PRACTICAL PSYCHIATRY OF OLD AGE

Practical Psychiatry of Old Age

JOHN WATTIS and MICHAEL CHURCH

NEW YORK UNIVERSITY PRESS
Washington Square, New York

First published 1986 in the United States of America
by NEW YORK UNIVERSITY PRESS, Washington Square,
New York, N.Y. 10003.

Library of Congress Cataloging-in-Publication Data

Wattis, John P., 1949–
 Practical psychiatry of old age.

 Bibliography: p.
 Includes index.
 1. Geriatric psychiatry. 2. Geriatric psychiatry–
Case studies. I. Church, Mike, 1953–. II. Title.
RC451.4.A5W38 1986   618.97′689   86-5291
ISBN 0-8147-9215-4

Printed and bound in Great Britain

CONTENTS

FOREWORD

In Britain at least two million, probably more, old people have significant mental disorders, and in a huge country like the United States the numbers are even greater. Apart from their own suffering, there is that of relatives and others upon whom their illnesses impinge. And then there is the army of people in the health and social services — general practitioners, nurses, social workers, remedial staff, psychologists and many others — who become involved during the course of their work. More and more of them are making this work their special concern, as members of the teams which form the specialist old age psychiatry services which are now established in many areas. The pressing demand for education in this field is visible everywhere. Lectures and courses are usually oversubscribed, and participants ask for advice about what to read. This book will be high among those I shall be recommending.

When he came to join us in Nottingham, John Wattis was the first full-time university lecturer in the psychiatry of old age in Britain. He brought with him many talents: a flair for communication; and a gift both for getting on with people, and for getting on with the job. This ability to collaborate is reflected not only in the emphasis of this book, but in its successful joint authorship. Mike Church belongs to a profession the rich potential contribution of which to the field of geriatric psychiatry has still to be fully realised, and this book should give that process a boost.

A new introductory book to the rapidly growing field of old age psychiatry is welcome. There is sufficient detail and technical material here for intelligent people of all professions to get their teeth into, but it should not go beyond the understanding of any; and it presents well the many-sided practical and humane approach which is characteristic of its authors and of the developing specialty itself.

In the eight years since he came to work with us in Nottingham, John Wattis has become, through successive national surveys, the main recorder and archivist of our field. Having completed his training he moved on to start a service of his own in Leeds, an enterprise mounted in a time of economic difficulty, yet he has won golden opinions from all who know his work. He is Secretary of the Specialist Section on Old Age in the Royal College of Psychiatrists. That on top of all this he has found time to produce with his former colleague Mike Church this excellent little textbook, illustrates well his talent for getting on with

vii

things. Readers of this book will find themselves better informed, and infected with the authors' enthusiasm.

Tom Arie, MA BM FRCP FRCPsych FFCM,
Professor of Health Care of the Elderly,
University of Nottingham

PREFACE

The possibility of this book was first suggested by Tom Arie, Professor of Health Care of the Elderly at the University of Nottingham, some years ago. The authors, who come from the different, but closely related, disciplines of psychiatry and psychology, subsequently worked together in the pioneering years of a new specialist psychiatric unit for the elderly in Leeds. During our period of close clinical and academic co-operation, we became aware of the need for a basic text for the practical approach to the psychiatric care of old people in a multidisciplinary setting. We wanted to write this, as far as possible, in non-technical language, that would make it accessible to a wide range of health and social care workers, and their trainees, and to the interested non-professional worker. Above all, we wanted to show quite clearly that if approached logically and with adequate resources, most of the psychological problems of old age could be ameliorated or resolved.

Throughout the text we have used the terms 'patient' and 'client' interchangeably. The people we serve are the same whatever we call them! We have also, for greater convenience, generally referred to patients in the female gender, since this reflects the fact that more women than men survive into old age.

We have ordered the book so that the basic background information and skills in approaching the problems of old age are dealt with first. Then, using a problem-solving approach, we have dealt with the different symptoms that old people present to doctors, nurses, psychologists and others. Finally, we have dealt in more detail with approaches to management, stressing the importance of considering elderly patients as whole people interacting with their environments. We have sprinkled our account liberally with case-histories, as we believe this is the only way to do justice to the complexity of the situations faced in real life. At the same time, especially in preparing flow charts and other figures to summarise the work, we are aware that we have sometimes over-simplified. We have provided references for those who wish to pursue topics at greater depth.

We are indebted to the Medical Illustration Departments at our respective hospitals, to our secretaries, and especially to the colleagues of all disciplines who have in one way or another contributed to the development of this work. Our thanks are also due to the journal *Geriatric*

Medicine which has been proving ground for many of the ideas developed in this text. Our hope is that this book will provide an enjoyable and informative read, but at the same time that it will be a useful reference work for the busy practitioner, of whichever discipline.

1 INTRODUCTION

The psychiatric care of old people is intellectually stimulating and emotionally rewarding. Nevertheless many professionals in the health field feel overwhelmed by the problems of mental illness in old people. It is true that the health and social services of the developed Western nations are under constant pressure from the increasing number of old people in their populations. Families, often without adequate support from statutory services, are cracking under the strain of caring for severely disabled old people. Residential and hospital facilities for those who need 24-hour care are often inadequate in quantity and quality. Most of all, many people, even workers in the field, are still beguiled by the myth of 'senility' and the attitude that 'nothing can be done'. Our generation is the first in modern history to face the challenge of having a relatively high proportion of elderly people. The rise in the elderly population has been largely as a result of successful public health measures. In poorer countries, infant mortality can still result in the death of half of all children born before they reach the age of five years. Malnutrition and the diseases of poverty then produce a constant attrition of the population so that very few survive into old age. It is largely because of the success of preventative medicine and falling birth rates, that the developed nations now face the need to plan improved health services for old people.[1] Table 1.1 illustrates how the number of over-65-year-old people in the British Isles has risen from about 5 per cent of the population at the turn of the century to around 15 per cent now. In Britain and other northwestern European countries the increase in the over-65-year-old population has more or less evened out, but an increase is forecast in the population of very elderly people. Table 1.1 also gives the proportion of people in the 75–84 and 85-years-and-over age groups. The very old are also the group who are most likely to suffer from physical or mental disability and social disadvantage. Table 1.2 gives the age-specific prevalence rates for dementia in old age found in an epidemiological study in Newcastle.[2] The prevalence rate of dementia in the oldest age group at around one in five is extremely high. Research evidence is beginning to accumulate that dementia in the very elderly may be a more benign process than in the young elderly. Nevertheless, the coincidence of high prevalence of dementia with a high prevalence of incapacitating physical disease and the fact that many very

1

old people live alone means that this group is particularly vulnerable, and particularly likely to need hospital care.

Table 1.1: Old People as a Percentage of the Total Population (UK)

	Over 65	75–84 years	85 years and over
1901	4.7	1.2	0.2
1951	11.0	3.1	0.5
1981	15.1	4.8	1.0
2001	14.3	5.0	1.5

Source: Adapted from *Dementia in Old Age.*[1]

Table 1.2: Age specific Prevalence Rates of Dementia (Newcastle Study)

Age	Percentage of 'chronic brain syndrome'
65–69	2
70–74	3
75–79	6
80 +	22

Source: Kay, Bergman, Foster, McKechnie and Roth (1970).[2]

Another way of looking at this is to consider the number of people in middle life who might be available to support the elderly. In England and Wales in 1931 there were more than ten people aged 45 to 64 years for each person aged 75 years and over. By 1951 this ratio had dropped to seven to one. In 1979 it was just over four to one and by 1991 it is estimated that it will only be around three to one. Despite good intentions, it is therefore likely that care of the elderly will have to depend more on organised provision and less on families. In the past, women have been the principal care-givers within most families but increased geographical dispersion of families as people seek for work, the rising number of women who work outside the house, the increasing number of one-parent families and women's own changing ideas of their role in life all mean that care is going to have to be shared more fairly around the community and not simply laid on the shoulders of a convenient member of the patient's family.

The northwestern European populations have been described by one demographer[3] as 'aged' but North America, the Soviet Union, Japan, Australia and most of southern and eastern Europe (the 'ageing populations') are still going through the phase of expansion in the 65–74-year-old group that northwestern Europe has already experienced. In the USA, for example, only 11 per cent of the population were aged 65 and over in 1980, rising to a projected 12 per cent in 1990 and 17 percent in 2030. These 'ageing' societies will probably go through the same kind of increase in the population of very old people as has already started to happen in northwestern Europe but at a later time. The developing countries at present have a much lower population of old people (e.g. southern Asia in 1975 had nearly one-third of the total world population, but only 14 per cent of those aged over 75 and over compared with Europe with 12 per cent of the total population, and 28 per cent of those aged 75 and over[3]).

In addition to international variations in the proportion of old people in populations, there are also local variations in the proportion of old people in different areas of each country, variations in survival by sex, and variations in the proportion of old people living alone or in institutions. In both the aged and ageing societies there is a tendency for the young people to migrate out of city centres and rural areas into suburbia. Some areas like the South Coast of Britain, and Florida in the USA, attract old people, who often move there on retirement. Florida, for example, has 18 per cent elderly, compared with the national rate of about 11 per cent in the USA. Old people in the UK and USA also share a tendency to be relatively poor and to live in poor accommodation. The United Kingdom is certainly one of the first countries to experience the ageing of its population, and because of the National Health Service is often seen as being amongst the world leaders in provision for the elderly. It is also the country in which both authors practise. We will therefore often describe the situation in our own community, qualifying this by reference to experience in other countries where this seems specially appropriate.

Psychiatric Services for Old People

In the face of all these statistics, it is tempting to give up and say 'nothing can be done'. The number of old people with dementia far exceeds the capacity of hospitals and old people's homes. Only about 5 or 6 per cent of the elderly are in any form of institutional care (Table 1.3) and a small shift of the elderly population into hospital care could easily swamp the system. The idea of the specialist psychiatrist as some kind of human furniture remover who is called in to arrange 'removal and storage' of the demented elderly person is outdated. Special psychiatric services for old people have demonstrated what can be done by proper assessment and management of mentally ill old people in the community. Old people do get a raw deal when it comes to public spending on their health and welfare and they are often too poor to buy adequate private services for themselves. Generally, in the UK, they are not organised as a political pressure group and it is easy for their needs to be ignored. In the USA, older Americans have been more vociferous. Political pressure is needed to improve spending on health and social care of old people but in this book we aim to show that intelligent application of existing resources can, by using them more efficiently, bring great benefit to older people and their relatives.

Table 1.3: Where Old People Live (England, 1976)

With spouse in two-person household	41%
Alone	28%
In other types of household	13%
With children	12%
In residential/hospital accommodation	6%

Source: Adapted from *Dementia in Old Age.*

Although the increase in the elderly population and in the prevalence of dementia has been the primary reason for the development of special psychiatric services for old people, there are other good reasons for their evolution. The presentation and management of mental disorders is different in old age. Leaving aside any spiritual dimension, the human organism can be seen largely as a group of physiological and anatomical systems designed to provide a constant environment for the brain, and to enact its orders. The ageing brain, however, seems to have less 'reserve' than in younger people and the supporting physiological systems are also often less able to cope with outside insults. For example, old people seem to be more susceptible to the toxic effects of general illnesses such as pneumonia and transient confusion is readily produced by such illnesses. Physical illness is also associated with depressed mood in many old people. Another reason for the different presentation and management of mental illness in old age is the different social background. The proportion of old people living alone is high (Table 1.3). With increasing age, this becomes more pronounced; half of all women in the UK over 75 years of age live alone.[4] Old people are also more often subjected to the stresses of bereavement. 'Young elderly' people sometimes find the burden of retirement hard to bear, especially when pensions are low. Old people are also more likely to live in substandard accommodation with poor sanitary facilities.

Co-operation between psychiatrists and physicians in geriatric medicine is vital. At a local level, this means that psychiatrists and physicians must be willing to respect each other's expertise, and co-operate in managing patients with mixed problems. Sometimes a patient with a psychiatric disorder may also need substantial geriatric care, and vice versa. If the patient needs inpatient care this can be on a joint ward. Nationally, few of these wards exist,[5] and when psychiatrists and physicians for the elderly have their beds on the same campus, they may not be needed. When physicians and psychiatrists work closely together they can decide on which ward a patient can best receive the care she needs.

Case 1.1:

> G.D. was an 80-year-old widow who lived alone. She was obese and had bilateral osteoarthritis of the hips. Her closest son had died tragically about three years before her first referral with depressive illness. On this occasion, she made a satisfactory, though not complete, response to antidepressant treatment. A year later she was referred again to the psychiatrist. She had taken to her bed, first locking the door, and refused to answer the phone. She was unable to get out of bed because her arthritis did not permit her to bend at the hip. She admitted to feeling depressed but attributed this to her loss of mobility. She did not show any signs at this stage of a severe depressive illness. A colleague in geriatric medicine agreed to admit her for mobilisation, and she cheered up as soon as she went to hospital. She was mobilised, and returned home within a few weeks. Immediately, she took to her bed, and the psychiatrist was called. He agreed to admit her and although she again made an initial response to hospitalisation and antidepressants, within a few weeks she became more overtly depressed and less mobile.

> We decided to start her on electroconvulsive therapy (ECT) for her depression but by this time, despite the best efforts of our psychiatric nurses, she was in danger of developing severe pressure sores. The physician in geriatric medicine agreed to take her to his ward for physical care, but it was arranged that she should attend the psychiatric department for ECT from the geriatric ward.

This kind of practical co-operation requires good relationships and a good understanding of the issues involved. To try to further this, the Royal College of Psychiatrists and the British Geriatrics Society agreed joint guidelines, published in 1979.[6] These were framed to ensure that there were no demarcation disputes between specialist medical and psychiatric services, and to ensure that paramount importance was given to the assessed needs of the patient.

There are no such professional guidelines for collaboration between social and medical services but in many localities fruitful practical co-operation has grown up with the understanding that despite gross short-ages of resources, both psychiatrists and social workers are trying to achieve what is best for their patients and clients.

The interaction of physical, psychiatric and social problems in old age and the consequent need for close co-operation between psychiatrists, geriatricians, nurses, social workers, clinical psychologists and other disciplines has influenced the evolution of specialist psychiatric services. This evolution has been a relatively recent affair. It has not been easy to document in the UK, as the Department of Health and Social Security does not recognise psychiatry of old age as a separate sub-speciality for statistical purposes. However, a survey conducted in 1980 to 1981[5] estimated that there were around 120 consultant psychiatrists working wholly or substantially in old age psychiatry in the United Kingdom. Over half of them were believed to have come to work in the area over the five years before the survey. By 1984, there were an estimated 150 to 160 consultants working in the field; this reflected a substantial increase during a period when the health service has not seen much overall growth. The 1981 survey showed that three-quarters of specialist services provided 'comprehensive' care for all psychiatric disorders in the elderly in a defined catchment area. About a tenth of services dealt only with demented people and the remainder were a mixture of 'comprehensive' and 'dementia' services. Most patients referred to psychiatric services for old people were inititally seen in their own homes by a consultant but a fifth of initial visits were carried out by other disciplines (mostly community nurses or social workers). Only a tenth of new referrals were initially seen in the outpatients department and fewer than one in twenty patients were admitted directly to inpatient facilities without any prior assessment. Most services were working with fewer facilities than those recommended by the Department of Health and Social Security ten years previously. These recommendations were, in any case, based on the over-65-year-old population and took no account of the continuing increase in the proportion of very old people. Despite recent advances, there are still many health districts in the United Kingdom without adequate psychogeriatric services and, sadly, a substantial minority without any specialist services at all.

Table 1.4 summarises some of the reasons for the development of specialist psychiatric services for old people. To these reasons perhaps could be added the need for local advocacy for mentally ill old people within health service planning. There seems little doubt that a consultant psychiatrist with special responsibility for old people acts as a focus for the development of services.

Table 1.4: Reasons for the Development of Specialist Services

1. Increasing number of old and very old people in the community
2. Prevalence of dementia in old people
3. Different presentation and management of disease in old people
4. Need for co-ordination of services and multidisciplinary working

Planning a Psychiatric Service for Old People

The functions of a comprehensive psychiatric service for old people can be broken down into four compartments. Assessment, meaning a comprehensive evaluation of the person's physical, psychiatric and social needs, should be thorough at the point of entry to the system and whenever a move from one compartment of care to another is envisaged. This model is illustrated in Figure 1.1. Systems which have inadequate assessment may, for example, provide expensive long-term care for people who, had they been adequately assessed, might only have needed a short period of medical treatment. Systems with inadequate acute or long stay institutional care may throw undue strain on staff involved in community treatment and support. As these staff are, or often should be, involved in assessment, this strain may further compromise the assessment function, perhaps leading to a breakdown in the whole system. Weakness in community support facilities can overload acute inpatient facilities and lack of long stay care can block exit from the acute inpatient facilities. In planning, therefore, the whole assessment, treatment and support network must be seen as an interactive system.

Figure 1.1: Functions of a Psychiatric Service for Old People

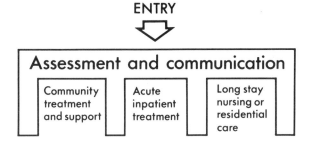

ENTRY

Assessment and communication

| Community treatment and support | Acute inpatient treatment | Long stay nursing or residential care |

The first essential in planning is to be clear about the 'target population'. In the UK it is reckoned that one consultant and the associated team of workers can cope effectively with an area containing about 22,000 old people.[8] With the increasing proprotion of very old people, that number should be reduced. In addition, in teaching health districts, where staff have responsibilities for under-graduate and post-graduate teaching, the catchment area should be cut to about 14,000 old people. A restricted geographical area is usually chosen because this enables the team to build up relationships with local general practitioners, district nurses, social workers, home helps and other social and voluntary services. The total population served must also be known in order to decide what personnel and facilities (for example, day hospital places and inpatient beds) are needed. Care of the elderly is an area where the traditional distinction between 'primary care' and hospital-based care is inadequate. In fact, the true 'primary carers' are not the general practitioner and area social worker but the family and neighbours of the affected person. The general practitioner and area social workers then act as the first line of statutory services but with the increasing emphasis on community care by hospital-based services, the old idea that care in the community was entirely the prerogative of the general practitioner needs to be re-evaluated. The hospital-based psychiatrist is much more than just a 'gate keeper' for admission to inpatient or day hospital facilities. The specialist team needs to work in co-operation with general practitioners and area social workers to set up adequate networks of care for the psychiatrically ill elderly in the community.

The typical specialist team consists of a consultant and one or more doctors in training as well as community nurses and social workers. In addition, there are likely to be occupational therapists, sometimes working across inpatient,day patient and community care, and physiotherapists. There are the nursing staff for the wards and day hospitals and many teams have some access to a clinical psychologist although few are fortunate enough to have one as a full-time member of the team. Access to speech therapists and other specialist workers varies from health district to health district. Inequalities in health care from one place to another are nowhere more evident than in the field of specialist psychiatric services for old people.

The best team in the world can do little if not backed by appropriate facilities. In the UK, the Royal College of Psychiatrists[8] and the Department of Health and Social Security[9] have both suggested guidelines for psychiatric services for the elderly and the Health Advisory Service has reiterated the former in its booklet 'The Rising Tide'.[10] Some of these guidelines are summarised in Table 1.5. The assessment and treatment beds are often located on one ward for all different types of mental illness although some services provide a separate ward for assessment of those who are markedly confused. The location of acute assessment beds is as important as their number. Because of frequent concurrent physical illness and the resultant need for ready access to laboratory and other investigative facilities and for close co-operation with geriatric medicine, these beds are best located on a district general hospital site. When they are so located, they can be used more efficiently. Unfortunately, many acute psychiatric facilities are still located in relatively remote mental hospitals although it has been government policy for a long time to move them into the district general hospital. The increasingly elderly population of many old institutions throws a great strain on nursing and other staff and militates against good standards of care.

Table 1.5: Guidelines for Special Provision for Mentally Ill Old People

Acute assessment and treatment beds	1.5 per 1,000 old people
Day hospital places (dementia and share of non-dementia places)	2.65–3.65 per 1,000 old people[a]
Long stay beds for demented old people	2.5–3 per 1,000 old people[b]

Sources: a. Royal College of Psychiatry.[8] b. Department of Health and Social Security.[9]

These hospitals are also where many of the long stay beds for elderly demented people are located. In this case, the problems are not access *to* diagnostic and geriatric medical services so much as access *for* elderly relatives and other visitors. This can lead to unhealthy isolation which robs the patient and staff of valuable contact with the outside community. Many wards in such institutions operate on very low staffing levels. In the heyday of the asylum system of care, there were many patients who were relatively able-bodied and able to contribute to the care of the more disabled patients. Now wards may have been halved in the number of patients they cater for but practically all their patients will be severely disabled and require a great deal of care. The development of acute psychiatric services and of specialised units has often meant that the 'long stay' wards where many of the elderly patients are concentrated have been relatively deprived of staff. The situation in the UK at present is very grave but moving patients out into smaller community-based units, although desirable, is expensive, especially as the dangerously low staffing levels of some large institutions cannot be sustained in smaller community units. Although the United Kingdom can be proud of its community diagnostic and caring services for old people, the standard of our institutional care falls below that of some other European countries.

The Department of Health and Social Security has produced and evaluated innovatory designs for community care of the mentally handicapped, and, if the money can be found, such designs could readily be adapted to the needs of mobile severely demented elderly people.

The recent increase in private care facilities in the UK, while it could be helpful, also poses several problems. First, old people generally do not get admitted to public institutions unless it can be demonstrated that they desperately need the care that can be provided in these institutions. There is no such 'filter' for admission to private care facilities and it is possible that such facilities may admit people who do not really 'need' the care they offer. Indeed, the commercial pressure would be to do just this, thereby keeping costs down, and profit margins up. Secondly, it has yet to be *demonstrated* that private care facilities cost less for the same level of care than do facilities provided by the National Health Service or the social services. There is in fact some suspicion that publically provided services may be more economical than private care. Thirdly, private care facilities can and sometimes do opt out of looking after residents who become disturbed, expecting the public sector services to take over difficult cases at a moment's notice. Finally, and despite the sterling work of the Health Advisory Service, this applies to public as well as private institutions, there is the need to develop a more effective means of monitoring standards of care and enforcing change where these are inadequate. Recent moves by the Department of Health and Social Security to establish a code of care[11] and monitoring by local health and social services authorities are a step in the right direction.

Day hospital facilities serve several different functions. Some places are used to support severely demented people whose relatives want to keep them at home but who need a regular 'break'. Others are used, perhaps inappropriately, to support those who are in need of 24-hour care while they wait for a place to become available in hospital or in a residential or nursing home. Another important group of users are those suffering from mental illnesses other than dementia. Many of these patients are suffering from depressive illness and day hospital treatment may avoid the need for inpatient care or may enable patients to be discharged home sooner and kept in relatively good health despite social isolation and other unfavourable circumstances. The effective functioning of day hospitals depends upon the provision of other facilities such as social services day centres. Transport is also a vital factor in day hospitals as most patients cannot make their own way to the hospital and transport services need to be arranged so that it is possible for them to wait a while for those who are not ready when the vehicle calls. Relatives, home helps, district nurses, community nurses and others need to be enlisted in many cases to make sure that the old person does attend the day hospital facility. Day hospitals whose primary function is assessment, treatment and rehabilitation are probably best located, together with acute beds, in the district general hospital. Day hospitals providing continuing support for the behaviourally disturbed demented could well be distributed with long stay beds throughout the community served. In some areas of relatively scattered populations, the 'mobile' day hospital has been evolved. Staff and equipment travel from the base hospital to a different location each day and run a day hospital in a local church hall, community centre or other suitable facility. This is a useful way of spreading thin resources across a wide geographical area.

The health care system in the USA is quite different. There is less emphasis on the 'primary care' function of general practitioners and private facilities provide much of the acute and continuing psychiatric care for old people. These are supported by private health insurance schemes, and for the poor, by complicated social security legislation. The net result is that the USA has some of the finest acute and long stay facilities in the world, but their availability is even more constrained by geographical and financial considerations than is the availablity of services in the UK. For a fuller discussion of the system of health care for the elderly in the USA and its funding the reader is referred to *The Core of Geriatric Medicine*.[12]

Social Services Provision

The vast majority of mentally ill old people live at home. If they are lonely or dependent for basic needs on others, then social services provision is often appropriate. Other forms of help have been recently added to the traditional pattern of home helps, meals-on-wheels and laundry services. The neighbourhood warden, who is paid by Social Services to provide a daily human contact for old people living alone, and family placement schemes where families are paid to take in old people, often to give their caring relatives a break, are two examples. Trained social workers are also beginning to take a greater interest in the personal needs of old people and their carers. Generally, at present most community services are only fully available from 9 a.m. to 5 p.m. five days a week. However, there is a need to experiment on the cost-effectiveness of extending these services to be more available at night and at weekends, as well as to evaluate the provision of special out-of-hours services such as night sitting. The systematic evaluation of alternative patterns of care has always been a weakness in Health and Social Services provision, and does not receive the attention it deserves from professional bodies and journals. We tend rather to provide services that seem a 'good idea' (if they are not too expensive) or even to provide services according to political dogma. This is not the way to be humane, effective, or efficient.

When old people need treatment, it is clearly the province of the general practitioner or the hospital authorities. When they need community services such as home help or meals-on-wheels, it is largely the responsibility of social services although district nurses and community psychiatric nurses often contribute. When patients need day care or 24-hour insititutional care, the position is not so clear. Theoretically, in the UK, people suffering from mild to moderate dementia with no serious associated physical illness receive social services residential care when needed, although the willingness of the social services department to take on responsibility for these people varies throughout the country. People with more severe dementia and a serious physical illness go to geriatric medical facilities when the family and local community can no longer keep them at home and people with severe dementia and 'behavioural' problems such as wandering or aggressiveness go to psychiatric long-term care. In practice, as several surveys have shown, there is an enormous overlap between levels of dependency in residential and hospital care.[13,14] This is partly because the increasing number of very old people with heavy and often mixed disability are the group in need of residential care and so tend to be admitted to such institutions. It is also because professionals working in this field sometimes feel it is cruel to move people whose 'home' is in residential care just because, with increasing age, their level of disability has increased beyond the theoretical 'upper limit'. The best solution might well be a combined care facility where staff were available to cope with all levels of disability. Someone admitted to such a facility would be able to stay there for the rest of their life and still get increased levels of nursing care should they need it. This is the pattern of care provided, for example, in some parts of Australia, where residential care facilities often have their own 'nursing home' on the same site. There has been no attempt to provide this kind of care systematically in the United Kingdom and the divided responsibilities with local authority housing departments or voluntary bodies responsible for sheltered housing, social services departments responsible for residential care and the National Health Service responsible for care of the more severely disabled, militates against it.

Voluntary Provision

Some of the finest initiatives in care of elderly people with psychiatric disorders are in the 'voluntary' sector. Housing associations provide sheltered housing which will often help alleviate the loneliness of the depressed old person or enable a husband/wife to continue looking after a demented spouse. Groups of relatives of elderly mentally ill people meet for mutual support and have even arranged informal day care facilities. Volunteers in 'good neighbour schemes' or 'care groups' do shopping or sit with elderly patients at home whilst relatives take a break. Some voluntary groups have even organised quite sophisticated day centres and work centres for old people which take their share of those with mental illness. In the USA and Australia voluntary and charitable bodies, often with church associations, have played a much more prominent role in developing nursing home, residential home and other facilities for long-term care and support of old people. Other schemes, such as the family placement scheme in Leeds, are organised by social services with payment to a family to take in old people usually for a few weeks at a time while the regular carers take a holiday.

Multidisciplinary Working

The involvement of different organisations and different disciplines in work for old people with mental illness provides an opportunity for creative co-operation if the workers and their respective organisations can get along together. If they cannot manage to do this, whole groups of elderly people can be left 'out in the cold' as health and social services dispute who is responsible. Most psychiatric services for old people are based on a team of people from different disciplines who, as well as providing services directly, also liaise with other workers in their own disciplines who are not direct members of the team. Patterns of working together vary widely from team to team and from time to time within a team. The following description illustrates how the team with which the authors are familiar functions at present. The method of dealing with

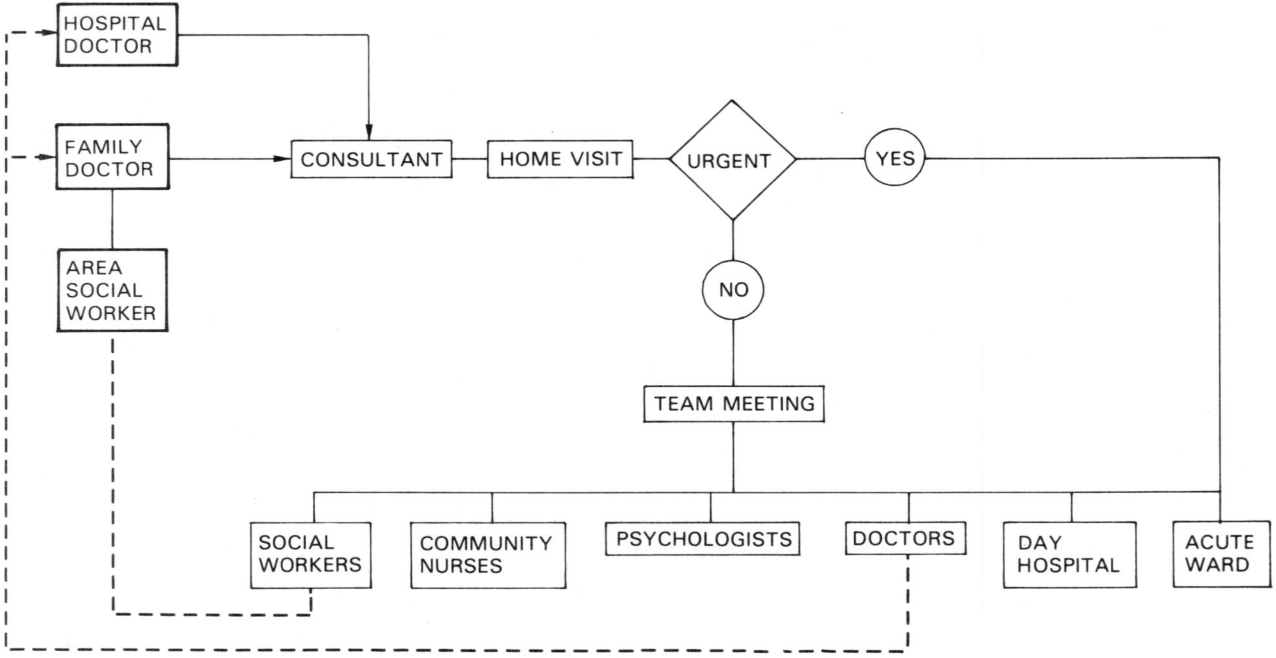

Figure 1.2: Flow Chart illustrating Working of a Particular Specialist Psychiatric Team

new referrals is illustrated in the flow chart in Figure 1.2. New referrals come, usually from the patient's family doctor (general practitioner), to the consultant or his secretary. Some referrals of inpatients come from hospital doctors and some 'community' referrals are really initiated by social workers with the approval of the appropriate general practitioner. Sometimes team members give informal advice to social workers or residential care staff about a particular problem without a referral being made. It is always made clear that this does not constitute a formal referral to the team and quite often the advice is that such a referral would be appropriate. Once a patient has been referred, he or she is seen at home by a senior member of the medical staff (consultant or senior registrar) and an initial assessment is made. This happens within 24 hours for urgent referrals and usually within a few days for less urgent cases. If the assessment indicates that urgent action is needed, the assessing doctor initiates this immediately. Otherwise the case is discussed at the weekly team meeting where the different disciplines have a chance to comment and make suggestions about management. Once a member of the team accepts responsibility for a particular patient in the community, that person becomes, regardless of discipline, the 'key worker' and is, as far as possible, the focus for any further management decisions. The team meeting also provides an opportunity for members of the team to present ongoing cases with whom they are having particular difficulties for group discussion and possibly to enlist the help of other disciplines in coping with the problem. Some patients are assessed to be in need of urgent medical rather than psychiatric attention. They are referred back to the family doctor or to the appropriate medical specialist (usually the physician in geriatric medicine). Many patients who are referred will be already known to local social workers who are invited to participate in meetings where their clients are to be reviewed and are generally kept in touch with how the team is managing their clients.

For successful multidisciplinary working, there has to be a sense of trust and mutual respect between team members. Because of the markedly different training between different disciplines, this can be hard to achieve. There are overlapping areas of expertise and it is only by discussing case management frankly in the multidisciplinary setting that the most appropriate skills can be applied to a particular patient's problems. One model for understanding the overlap between different disciplines is presented in Figure 1.3 Each discipline has its area of expertise. For example, area A in the doctor's portion of the figure represents such things as medical diagnosis and the prescribing of drugs where only the doctor has the appropriate training and skills. A similar area for the nurse might be the planned provision of 24-hour care to support patients and at the same time help them to develop their own self-care skills. For the social worker, detailed planning and provision of support services in the community might be a similar area. Other areas of skill and responsibility overlap (B). A simple example of this is the giving of injections where both doctors and nurses have appropriate training. Yet other areas (C) may be shared by all members of the team. All disciplines, for example, might have training in bereavement counselling. The diagram is over-simplified but still gives some idea of the complexity of multidisciplinary working. The psychologist on the team may have speical skills in neuro-psychological and behavioural assessment but will also share some skills in counselling or psychotherapy with other disciplines. The same mixture of unique and shared skills is also found in occupational therapy, physiotherapy and other disciplines. The exact areas of overlap in any team will depend not only on disciplinary boundaries, but also on individual training. What is important is that the areas of unique skill or responsibility and of overlap are recognised and that team members are prepared to accept each other's skills, regardless of different training backgrounds. Members of the team must also guard against the tendency to concentrate on the more 'interesting' aspects of work while the more mundane tasks are left undone, and be secure enough in their own work to listen to constructive criticism from other disciplines. If such an ethos can be achieved, mistakes in planning care will be minimised, as all members of the team are enabled to contribute responsibly.

Figure 1.3: Overlaps of Skill in the Multidisciplinary Team

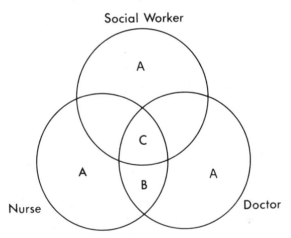

Another potential source of conflict in multidisciplinary working is the different hierarchical structure of different disciplines illustrated in Figure 1.4. This figure, again, is an over-simplification as only three disciplines are included. Medicine is the only discipline where authority rests more or less absolutely with the most senior clinical member of the team. Other disciplines have to rely, to varying degrees, on the decisions of more senior members of their disciplines who are not involved in the day-to-day clinical working of the team. If they have good higher managers who are prepared to delegate authority and the team members are able and willing to accept this, then everything can work well. If this delegation cannot be achieved, for whatever reason, true multidisciplinary working is hard to achieve.

Figure 1.4: Hierarchical Professional Structures and the Multidisciplinary Team

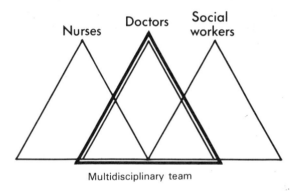

Multidisciplinary team

The Spectrum of Mental Disorder in Old Age

The classification of mental illness in old age will be discussed more fully in Chapter 3. However, at this stage, it is important to emphasise that not all mental disorder in old age is dementia. Epidemiological studies of the prevalence of mental disorder in old age are notoriously difficult to conduct. Even with relatively easily defined disorders like dementia and depressive psychosis, a considerable range of prevalence figures has been shown in different studies. Assumptions have also been made in the past that problems such as neurosis, personality disorders and alcoholism decrease with increasing age but recent evidence does not bear this out. The two main myths about mental disorder in old age which this book sets out to challenge are, first, that all mental illness in old age is dementia and, secondly, that 'nothing can be done' about mental illness in old age. In this chapter we have reviewed the increasing pressure on health and social services caused by the increasing number of old and especially very old people in our population. We have seen how the population pressures, the prevalence of dementia, the differences in other mental illnesses in old age and the need to focus action in multi-skilled and multidisciplinary teams, have led to the evolution of specialist psychiatric services for old people in many, but by no means all, health districts. We have briefly reviewed the setting up of such a team, the facilities it needs and how it relates to social services and voluntary provision for old people. We have also discussed some of the potential benefits and problems of multidisciplinary working. In Chapters 2 and 3 we discuss some of the skills needed by doctors and other disciplines in the assessment and management of elderly people with mental disorder. In Chapters 4 to 7 we discuss some of the main presentations of mental disorder in old age and these chapters are planned to be an easy source of reference for those confronted with these problems. In Chapters 8 to 10 we discuss in more detail some of the approaches to treatment of the elderly mentally ill, embracing, not only conventional medical treatment, but also a practical psychological approach to the individual sufferer, his family and environment.

Notes

1. Wells, N.E.J., *Dementia in Old Age* (Office of Health Econommics, London, 1979).

2. Kay, D.W.K., Bergmann, K., Foster E.M., McKechnie, A.A. and Roth, M. *Comprehensive Psychiatry*, 11, 1970, 26–35.

3. Grundy, E. , 'Demography and Old Age', *Journal of the American Geriatrics Society*, 31, 1983, 6, 325–32.

4. Hunt, A. The Elderly at Home. A survey carried out by the Social Survey Division of the Office of Population Censuses and Surveys on behalf of the Department of Health and Social Security, (HMSO, London, 1978).

5. Wattis, J., Wattis, L. and Arie, T. 'Psychogeriatrics: A National Survey of a New Branch of Psychiatry', *British Medical Journal*, 282, 1981, 1529–33.

6. British Geriatrics Society, and Royal College of Psychiatrists, 'Guidelines for Collaboration between Geriatric Physicians and Psychiatrists in the Care of the Elderly', *The Bulletin of the Royal College of Psychiatrists*, 1979, 168–9.

7. Wattis, J. and Arie, T. 'Further Developments in Psychogeriatrics in Britain', *British Medical Journal*, 289, 1984, 778.

8. Royal College of Psychiatrists, 'Interim Guidelines for Regional Advisors on Consultant Posts in the Psychiatry of Old Age', *The Bulletin of the Royal College of Psychiatrists*,

1981, 110–11.

9. Department of Health and Social Security, *Services for Mental Illness Related to Old Age,* HM(72)71 (1972).

10. Dick, D.H. *The Rising Tide: Developing Services for Mental Illness in Old Age* (NHS Health Advisory Service, Sutton, 1982).

11. *Home Life: A Code of Practice for Residential Care,* (Centre for Policy on Ageing, London, 1984).

12. Libow, L.S., Schechter, Z. and Margolis, E. 'Demographic and Economic Aspects' in L.S. Libow and F.T. Sherman, *The Core of Geriatric Medicine* (The C.V. Mosby Company, St Louis, Missouri, 1981).

13. Wilkin, D., Mashiah, T. and Jolley, D.J., 'Changes in Behavioural Characteristics of Elderly Populations in Local Authority Homes and Long Stay Hospital Wards 1976–77, *British Medical Journal,* 1978, 2, 1274–6.

14. Clarke, M.G., Williams, A.J. and Jones, P.A., 'A Psychogeriatric Survey of Old People's Homes', *British Medical Journal,* 283, 1981, 2, 1307–10.

2 PSYCHIATRIC AND PHYSICAL ASSESSMENT

The skills needed to assess and formulate the management of elderly patients are best developed in clinical practice and by review of outcome in individual patients. If we are to learn from this experience, we must be meticulous in recording our findings and opinions in individual cases and in comparing our initital impressions with outcome. The self-discipline of careful assessment, problem formulation and review of outcome is the foundation for professional growth. The scheme outlined here is intended as the framework for such learning.

History

Most elderly patients referred for psychiatric assessment should be seen initially in their own homes. The advantages of this practice hold true for family doctors and members of other disciplines and include:

1. The patient is seen in the situation with which he or she is familiar. The confusion and disorientation which may be engendered by a trip to hospital, general practice surgery or consulting rooms are avoided.
2. The environment can be assessed as well as the patient. Table 2.1 lists some of the important factors in assessment of the home.
3. The patient's function in his or her own environment and the level of social support can easily be assessed.
4. Neighbours and relatives are often readily available to give a history of the illness and its impact on them.

Elderly patients who have to be seen for the first time in hospital should be interviewed in a quiet, distraction-free environment, and every effort must be made to put them at their ease. It is quite impossible to conduct a satisfactory psychiatric assessment of an elderly person who may have poor sight or hearing or both in a ward environment where there is a lot of noise and distraction. Unless care is taken to make an assessment in a suitable environment, any confusion will be compounded and a falsely pessimistic opinion of the patient's mental function may be formed. The

20

Table 2.1: Assessment of the Home — Some Important Factors

General level of repair and tidiness of property
Who does the cooking/cleaning/shopping?
Heating, lighting and ventilation
Water supply
Toilet and bathing facilities
Cooking arrangements and food stocks
The stairs
Accident hazards
Sleeping arrangements: has the bed been slept in?
Bottles; other evidence of alcohol abuse

patient's family and neighbours often have an important role to play in assessment and continuing management. A good relationship with them as well as with the patient is essential. At the inital interview, the patient and family will have many different anxieties, some of which may be founded upon their own ideas about the purpose of the assessment. It is vital that the doctor spends time listening to the problems as they are seen by the patient and relatives. A popular misconception is that the doctor has come to 'put away' the patient in the local institution. Social workers may suffer from a similar problem in that elderly clients may think that the social worker has come to arrange for them to be taken into 'a home'. The elderly patient's idea of what institutional care involves may also be quite different from that of the person conducting the assessment. Old people still refer to what we think of as modern hospitals by their workhouse names and find it difficult to conceive that an admission to hospital or a residential home could be anything other than permanent. The doctor needs to take time to listen to these fears and to explain why he is visiting and the scope and limitations of any help he can offer. Anxiety may inhibit the patient's and relative's ability to grasp and remember what is being said. It may be necessary to repeat the same information several times and to ask the patient or relative questions to clarify whether they have really understood what has been said. Those of us who work in the health field should never forget that although an assessment may be commonplace to us, for the patient and relative it is taking place at a crisis point in life. An empathetic manner, reflecting back the patient's and relative's concerns, will help them to realise that their worries have been acknowledged and will help to form a useful relationship.

The psychiatric history starts with the presenting complaint. Quite often, the patient lacks insight and believes that nothing is wrong. In these circumstances, careful probing is appropriate. Even early in the interview it may sometimes be necessary to ask direct questions about memory loss, mood or persecutory ideas, though a more oblique approach starting with personal history is usually better. As well as delineating the presenting complaint, it is important to obtain a history of how long it has been present and how it developed. Sometimes, when it is difficult to obtain a clear history of the time course of an illness, it is useful to resort to 'time landmarks'. These are things like the previous Christmas or some important personal anniversary which can often help to clarify the picture. Often a proper history of the presenting complaint can only be obtained by talking to an informant. Sometimes one can arrange to talk to a relative before seeing the patient and this is often helpful. In other cases, there may be no relatives available and information may have to be pieced together from a variety of sources such as the home help, the social worker and friends and neighbours. After delineating the presenting complaint and often even before this, it is helpful to get the patient to give an account of his previous life. Old people generally enjoy talking about the past and it is quite easy to introduce the subject. A useful opening line is 'tell me a bit about yourself; were you born in these parts?' One can then lead the person through their life history, often unobtrusively testing their memory (for example, their date of birth and the dates of important events) at the same time. The family history and the history of past physical and nervous complaints can be woven into this brief account of the patient's life-time and an assessment can be made of the patient's personality and characteristic ways of dealing with stress. Old people, like young people, respond well to those who have a genuine interest in them. Courtesy is also vital. Talking 'across' patients to other professionals or to relatives generates anxiety and resentment, as does lack of punctuality.

Mental State Examination

Level of Awareness

At an early stage in the interview, the patient's level of awareness should be assessed. The patient may be drowsy as a result of lack of sleep or medication or because of physcial illness. Rapidly fluctuating level of awareness is seen in acute confusional states and a level of awareness that fluctuates from day to day is one of the clues to the diagnosis of chronic subdural haematoma. Impaired awareness can lead to poor function on tests of cognition and memory and, if it is not recognised, can lead to an under-estimation of the patient's true abilities. The patient's ability to *concentrate* and pay *attention* are closely related to level of awareness. Sometimes, however, they may be distracted by more mundane things. If the patient is, for example, in pain, it may be very hard for him to understand the relevance of giving an account of his mental state. Disturbance of mood and abnormal perceptual experiences can also impair attention and concentration.

Behaviour

On a home visit the patient's behaviour can not only be observed directly but can also be deduced from the state of the house (see Table 2.1). The patient's general appearance, his dress, personal hygiene and the attitude to the interviewer can all be assessed. Incontinence can often be smelled and the patient's mobility checked by asking him to walk a few steps. Especially if the patient lives alone, inconsistencies between the patient's state and the state of cleanliness and organisation of the household indicate either that there is a good active social support network or that the patient has deteriorated over a relatively short period of time. There are available various behavoural schedules which enable the systematic assessment of the patient's abilities. A shortened form of the Crighton Royal Behavioural Assessment Form is shown in Table 2.2. It enables a numerical value to be attached to a person's performance in various important areas of behaviour. The advantages of such a scale are that it reminds the assessor of important areas and it enables discrepancies between different areas of performance to be highlighted so that potentially treatable problems are easily seen and dealt with. It also enables a ready comparison between different patients and between the same patients at different points in time even when the assessment is made by a different person. Finally, it gives an overall rating of disability which can be used to predict whether or not a patient is in need of a particular kind of institutional care. There are many such scales[1] and they are all imperfect but they do at least enable a systematic approach to the assessment of behaviour and they are usually extremely quick to fill out. Another form which could be recommended is the behavioural assessment form of the Clifton Assessment Procedure for the Elderly[2] (for discussion of this see Chapter 9). This has been applied to a wide range of patients in their own homes, in hospital and in other institutional settings and also measures overall levels of disability.

Mood or Affect

Mood in the technical sense used by psychiatrists is more than just how we feel. It has been described as 'a complex background state of the

Table 2.2: Modified Crighton Royal Behavioural Scale

Dimension		Score
MOBILITY	Fully ambulant including stairs	0
	Usually independent	1
	Walks with minimal supervision	2
	Walks only with physical assistance	3
	Bed-fast or chair-fast	4
ORIENTATION	Complete	0
	Orientated in ward, identifies persons correctly	1
	Misidentifies persons but can find way about	2
	Cannot find way to bed or toilet without assistance	3
	Completely lost	4
COMMUNICATION	Always clear, retains information	0
	Can indicate needs, understands simple verbal directions, can deal with simple information	1
	Understands simple information, cannot indicate needs	2
	Cannot understand information, retains some expressive ability	3
	No effective contact	4
CO-OPERATION	Actively co-operative, i.e. initiates helpful activity	0
	Passively co-operative	1
	Requires frequent encouragement or persuasion	2
	Rejects assistance, shows independent but ill-directed activity	3
	Completely resistive or withdrawn	4
RESTLESSNESS	None	0
	Intermittent	1
	Persistent by day	2
	Persistent by day, with frequent nocturnal restlessness	3
	Constant	4
DRESSING	Correct	0
	Imperfect but adequate	1
	Adequate with minimum of supervision	2
	Inadequate unless continually supervised	3
	Unable to dress or retain clothing	4
FEEDING	Correct, unaided at appropriate times	0
	Adequate, with minimum supervision	1
	Inadequate unless continually supervised	2
	Needs to be fed	3
CONTINENCE	Full control	0
	Occasional accidents	1
	Contintent by day only if regularly toileted	2
	Urinary incontinence in spite of regular toileting	3
	Regular or frequent double incontinence	4

organism' and, although this is rather an elaborate definition, it reminds us that mood affects not only how we feel but also how we think and even the functioning of our motor and gastro-intestinal systems. Old people are not always used to talking about their feelings and it can sometimes be quite difficult to find the right words. 'How do you feel in your spirits?' can evoke the appropriate response but will sometimes produce an account of the patient's alcohol drinking behaviour! Especially where there are communciation difficulties, one may have to resort to direct questioning, for example 'do you feel happy or sad?' Although the patient's account of her mood should always be sought, it cannot always be relied upon. Some elderly patients who are quite depressed, even to the point of being in tears throughout the interview, do not confess to a depressed mood, perhaps because they are afraid this may result in hospitalisation. Psychomotor retardation (the slowing of thought and action) can be so profound that patients are unable to report their mood or may even say 'I feel nothing.' The person conducting the assessment will, of course, observe the patient's facial expression, any tears and other signs of depressed mood. In addition, specific questions should be asked about whether the patient feels guilty about anything, whether they have any worries about money or health and, if there is depressed mood, enquiry should also be made in all cases about suicidal feelings. This can easily be introduced in a non-threatening way by a phrase such as 'have you ever felt that life was not worth living?' If the patient responds positively to this, further probes can then be made about ideas of self-harm. The risk of suicide must always be taken very seriously in old people who are depressed; depressed elderly men living alone, especially in the time following a bereavement, are particularly at risk. Often, if psychomotor retardation is present, the answer will take some time to come and it is very easy to rush on to the next question before the patient has had time to respond to the previous one. One group of symptoms is often associated with severe 'biological' depression. This includes early morning wakening, mood worse in the morning and profound appetite loss and weight loss. The opposite of depressed mood is elated mood which is seen in hypomania. The younger hypomanic patient is characterised by infectious good humour and feelings of happiness and impatience with those around him who do not share in his great plans for the world. In older patients, irritability and querulousness are often more prominent than happiness although the patient may still experience a feeling of elation and special powers.

Anxiety is felt by many elderly patients, often in response to the stresses of ageing. Sometimes the patient may be so worried about falling that, in order to avoid anxiety, she restricts her life severely. Thus, a patient who has had one or two falls may, instead of seeking medical help, restrict herself to a downstairs room in the house and never go out. As long as the patient continues to restrict her life, she experiences little anxiety. Whereas in a young person such behaviour would almost certainly lead immediately to the patient being defined as 'sick' and a call for medical attention, in the elderly patient, this restriction is all too easily accepted as 'normal'. When assessing anxiety, attention should therefore be paid not only to how the patient is feeling during the interview (which may, in itself, provoke anxiety!) but also to whether he or she can engage in the tasks of daily living without experiencing undue anxiety. Anxiety is an effect which has physiological accompaniments; a racing pulse, 'palpitations', 'butterflies in the stomach', sweating and diarrhoea are all found. Patients not infrequently use the term 'dizziness' to describe not true vertigo, but a feeling of unreality associated with severe anxiety. Sometimes the physiological changes induced by overbreathing, such as tingling in the arms and even spasm of the muscles of the hand and arm, may make matters worse.

Perplexity is the feeling which commonly accompanies acute confusional states and may also be found in some mildly demented patients. The patient in an acute confusional state may be experiencing visual or auditory hallucinations and may also be subjected to a whole series of changes in the environment which she cannot properly grasp. The human organism is always trying to make sense of its surroundings and so it is not surprising that patients in this sort of position feel perplexed. It is an effect that is not often described but it is a useful diagnostic pointer for acute confusional states. The puzzlement ('delusional mood') experienced by some patients early in a schizophrenic illness in some ways resembles the perplexity found in acute confusion, but the other characteristics of acute confusional states (e.g. fluctuating awareness and physical illness) usually make the distinction clear.

Thought

The form, speed and content of thought are all assessed. Formal thought disorder occurs in schizophrenia and includes thought-blocking when the patient's thoughts come to an abrupt end, thought withdrawal when thoughts are felt to be withdrawn from the patient's head, and thought insertion. For fuller description of these phenomena, the reader is referred to a standard text-book of psychiatry.[3] Slowing of the stream of thought (thought retardation) is found in many depressive disorders. Slow thinking is also characteristic of some of the organic brain syndromes caused by metabolic deficiencies. Thought is speeded up in hypomania, often leading to 'flight of ideas' where one thought is built upon another in a way that is founded upon tenuous associations. The patient with flight of ideas can be seen to have a logical thread running through their thoughts even if the subject develops and changes rather rapidly. In dementia, spontaneous thought is often diminished, so-called 'poverty of thought'. The patient with an acute confusional state also finds difficulty in maintaining a train of thought due to fluctuating awareness. In dementias of metabolic origin and in some cases of multi-infarct dementia, slowing of thought processes may be accompanied by great difficulty in assembling the necessary knowledge to solve particular problems. The observer gets the impression that the patient grasps what the problem is but is frustrated by her own inability to cope with it. Content of thought is profoundly influenced by the patient's mood. The depressed patient will often have very gloomy thoughts and ideas of poverty, or physical illness may be pervasive. The anxious patient's thoughts may be taken up with how to avoid various anxiety-provoking situations and there may be unnecessary worries about all aspects of everyday living. This kind of anxiety is also found in depressed patients, particularly if their normal personalities incline towards anxiety. The patient who feels persecuted may think of little else. Every noise or happening will be fitted into the persecutory framework. Except when patients are deeply suspicious, their *talk* generally reflects their thought. In addition, however, to the form, speed and content of thought, talk is also influenced by various motor functions. Slurred speech may be found in the patient who is drowsy or under the influence of drugs or alcohol. Sometimes it also results from specific neurological problems such as a stroke. Patients with Parkinson's disease may produce so-called 'scanning' speech where words are produced without inflexion and with hesitation between words. Patients with severe Parkinsonism may have difficulty in forming sounds at all. A degree of difficulty in finding words and putting speech together appropriately is found in many patients with dementia, particularly those with Alzheimer's disease. This is one form of dysphasia. A stream of apparent nonsense, so-called fluent dysphasia, may occur in dementia but is also sometimes associated with a small stroke. The general behaviour of the patient, which is not 'demented', and the sudden onset of the dysphasia, provide important diagnostic clues here. Occasionally, fluent dysphasia, especially when it includes new words 'invented' by the patient (neologisms) may be mistaken for the so-called 'word salad' produced by some schizophrenic patients. Again, the suddenness of onset and the absence of other signs of schizophrenia help in distinguishing these.

Hallucinations

These can be defined as perceptions without external objects. Visual hallucinations are usually seen in patients with acute confusional states or dementia although occasionally they occur in patients with very poor eyesight without measurable organic brain damage, especially if the patient is living alone in a relatively under-stimulating environment. Auditory hallucinations (hearing voices) occur in a variety of mental illnesses. They are predominantly found in schizophrenia when they may consist of a voice repeating the patient's thoughts or of voices talking about the patient in the third person. They also occur in severe depressive illness when they are often derogatory in nature. In hypomania, too, auditory hallucinations in keeping with the patient's mood are sometimes found. Hallucinations of touch and smell also occur. Hallucinations of being touched, especially those with sexual connotations, occur in the late-onset form of schizophrenia ('late paraphrenia') and hallucinations of smell, especially of the patient believing herself to smell 'rotten', in severe depression.

Delusions

A delusion can be defined as a false unshakeable belief out of keeping with the patient's cultural background. Delusions occur in fragmentary forms in organic mental states but well-developed delusions are usually found only in severe affective disorders and schizophrenia. The ideas of poverty, guilt or illness found in the less severely depressed patient may develop into absolute convictions in the more severely depressed. The patient may, for example, firmly believe that she has cancer in the face of all available medical evidence. Occasionally, of course, she will be right but in many cases the belief will be founded upon the depressed mood and will disappear when that is treated. Ideas of persecution are also sometimes found in patients with depression of moderate severity and these, too, can develop into full-blown delusions. This can make the differential diagnosis of atypical affective states and paraphrenia particularly difficult in old age. Delusions of grandeur, for example that the patient has extraordinary powers of perception or is fabulously rich, are also found in hypomanic states. In paranoid schizophrenia, the delusional content is often very complicated and may involve persecutory activities by whole groups of people. These delusions may be supported by hallucinatory experiences.

Obsessions and Compulsions

Obsessions occur when the patient feels compelled to repeat the same thought over and over again. They can be distinguished from schizophrenic phenomena such as thought insertion by the fact that obsessional patients feel that these thoughts come from within themselves and try to resist them. Sometimes such thoughts may result in compulsive actions, for example, returning many times to check that the door has been locked. Although characteristically a part of obsessional neuroses, obsessional symptoms also occur in depressed patients and apparently compulsive behaviour can also be a result of memory loss. Some patients, for example, with early dementia may not be able to remember that they have locked the door so may return many times to check it but not as a result of any inner feelings of compulsion.

Illusions

Illusions occur when a patient misinterprets a real perception. Some hypochondriacal worries can be based on this. For example, many old people have various aches and pains but sometimes patients may become over-concerned by these and may begin to worry that they indicate some physical illness. Such misinterpretations of internal perceptions are not usually described as illusions although the term would be quite appropriate. Acute confusional states also produce illusions when the patient, seeing the doctor approaching, misinterprets this as someone coming to do him harm and strikes out. This kind of misinterpretation can often be avoided as described by appropriate management (see Chapters 5 and 9).

Orientation/Memory

Orientation for time, place and person should be recorded in a systematic way. The degree of detail would depend upon the time available and the purpose of the examination. Orientation for time can easily be split into gross orientation, for example, the year or approximate time of day (morning, afternoon, evening, night), and finer orientation, for example, the month, the day of the week and the hour of the day. Orientation for person depends upon the familiarity of the person chosen as a point of reference. Orientation for place also depends upon familiarity. A useful brief scale which includes some items of orientation as well as some items of memory-testing is the scale developed by Hodkinson[4] from a longer scale which has been previously correlated with a degree of brain pathology in demented patients.[5] The Hodkinson Memory Information Scale is reproduced in Table 2.3.

Orientation is, to a large extent, dependent upon memory although it should never be forgotten that the patient may not know the name of the hospital she is in, simply because she has never been told. Memory for remote events can be assessed when taking the patient's history. The ability to encode new material can be assessed by the capacity to

Table 2.3: 10-Item Memory-information Score (Hodkinson, (1972))[4]

1.	Age
2.	Time (to nearest hour)
3.	Address for recall at end of test — this should be repeated by the patient to ensure that it has been heard correctly: 42 West Street
4.	Year
5.	Name of hospital (place seen)
6.	Recognition of two people
7.	Date of birth
8.	Years of First World War
9.	Name of present monarch
10.	Count backwards 20–1

remember a short address or to remember the interviewer's name. Many patients with dementia will have great difficulty in encoding and storing new memories. Sometimes, especially in the metabolic dementias, one can form the impression that the patient is encoding and storing new material but that they are having great difficulty in retrieving the memory when asked to. This has been described as 'forgetfulness'.

Other Areas of Organic Brain Dysfunction

When a patient has impaired memory, it is important to ascertain whether this is an isolated deficit or whether it is associated with other signs of more generalised brain damage. The detailed localisation of neuro-psychological signs is a very complicated matter because of the inter-dependence of different areas of brain function. This issue is further discussed in Chapter 9. However, in everyday clinical practice, some areas are relatively easy to test and these are mentioned here. *Right/left orientation* can be ascertained by asking the patient to lift their right or left hand. More complicated tasks such as 'touch your left ear with your right hand' are more discriminating but also more difficult to interpret. *Visuospatial function* can easily be tested by asking the patient to copy designs of increasing complexity. In clinical practice, one of the authors usually asks the patient to copy in turn a square, a triangle and a simple house. This should be done on paper without lines. *Nominal aphasia* can be tested using everyday objects. An object such as a pen or wrist-watch and its smaller parts can be used. *Frontal signs* may be picked up when patients perseverate on some of the tasks given to them. They may get stuck, for example, on their date of birth, repeating their year of birth when asked the current year or their age. Apraxia and perseveration may also be seen in tasks of everday living such as dressing. One of the authors vividly recalls a patient who had such advanced perseveration that when she went up a flight of stairs she continued the climbing motion even when she reached the top. More detailed descriptions of organic mental state examination can be found in Lishman's *'Organic Psychiatry'*[6] and *Dementia: A Clinical Approach.*[7]

Insight and Judgement

In severe psychiatric illness insight is often lost. Depressed patients may be unable to accept that they will get better despite remembering many previous episodes of depression which have improved with treatment. Hypomanic and paraphrenic patients may act on their delusions with disastrous consequences. Patients with severe dementia often do not realise their plight, which is perhaps fortunate. Patients with milder dementia may have some insight, especially in the metabolic and multi-infarct types of dementia where mood is, not surprisingly, also often depressed. Closely related to insight is judgement. This can be a particularly difficult question with a moderately demented patient living alone or living with relatives but left alone for a substantial part of the day. Patients may be leaving gas taps on and frankly be dangerous to themselves and others but at the same time maintain that they are looking after themselves perfectly well and do not need any help, much less residential or nursing home care. In areas where standards of care are high they may also have a mistaken image of the care they are refusing. Cases like this call for careful professional judgement from experienced workers. When should the patient's own judgement be considered so impaired that it can be overridden? If a person is to be 'persuaded' to go into long-term institutional care, should compulsory powers be involved? Can a demented patient be said to be giving 'informed consent' to any treatment? When demented patients who are not compulsorily detained wander off the ward, is it appropriate to bring them back 'informally' but under protest or should the compulsory legal powers of formal detention be invoked? Common sense, professional judgement and inter-disciplinary consultation must be applied and it should be remembered that the compulsory legal powers are intended to protect patients, not make life unbearable for them and those looking after them. The 1983 Mental Health Act (UK) and some United States provisions are discussed in more detail in Chapter 10.

Other Cognitive Functions

Mental arithmetic is used to test cognitive ability. The patient's educational level should be taken into acount and tasks should be related to everyday tasks (e.g. shopping) whenever possible. Many British old people still find it easier to reckon up in pre-decimal coinage. Tasks like serially subtracting seven from one hundred assess concentration as well as arithmetic and may be seen as irrelevant by many old people. They should generally be avoided. Asking the meaning of *proverbs* is also said to test abstract reasoning ability. Such tests rarely reveal clinically useful material in old people.

A brief summary of mental state evaluation is given in Table 2.4. It has been put into a mnemonic form which can be useful in everyday clinical practice.

Table 2.4: Summary of Mental State Evaluation

Awareness	— level of consciousness, fluctuation, attention and concentration
Behaviour	— general appearance of the patient (and his house) as well as behaviour during interview. Standardised form.
Affect	— depression, elation, anxiety, perplexity. Suicide risk. Somatic changes (e.g. sleep pattern, constipation, appetite, weight loss in depression; palpitations, tremor, churning stomach in anxiety).
Thought and talk	— form, speed, content, dysarthria, dysphasia, perseveration
Hallucinations, delusions, obsessions, illusions	
Orientation	— time, place and person
Memory	— remote, ability to encode new information, forgetfulness
Apraxia	— in everyday tasks (e.g. dressing, feeding). Constructional tasks
Nominal aphasia	— everyday objects in order of increasing difficulty
Judgement and insight	
Other cognitive functions (e.g. arithmetic, proverbs)	
Educational level must be taken into account.	

The psychiatric history and examination of the elderly patient takes time. It must be tailored to the patient's tolerance of questions and must be approached in a sympathetic way. The doctor who initiates his interview by firing a series of seemingly random questions designed to test memory and orientation is unlikely to get the best out of his patient. Time taken in proper assessment is not wasted. A poor assessment can result in treatable illness going untreated or a potentially independent old person being forced into dependency in an institution.

Psychiatric illness in the elderly is often complicated or precipitated by acute or chronic physical illness. For this reason, specialists in the psychiatry of old age usually work closely with their colleagues in the medicine of old age.

Caird and Judge's book on assessment of the elderly patient[8] gives a detailed account of physical assessment which can be used to fill out the following brief outline. Figure 2.1 illustrates some of the ways in which physcial disease may be related to psychiatric disorder. It reminds us that medical treatment for psychiatric disorder can cause physical illness and vice versa. No psychiatric examination, particularly in the elderly, is complete without a thorough physical examination. This can be done in the patient's home, especially if one has the benefit of joint visiting with a community nurse. In many cases, it may be more appropriate to bring the patient to the outpatient clinic or the general practice surgery for this part of the examination. In outpatients, a joint psychiatric-geriatric clinic can facilitate the management of difficult cases.

Figure 2.1: Relationships between Physical Disease and Psychiatric Disorder

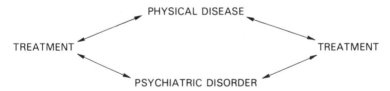

Diminished sensory input, one of the techniques used in 'brain washing', is often inflicted on the elderly due to medical slowness in recognising and correcting defects of sight and hearing. Sensory deprivation may be instrumental in producing paranoid states and in precipitating or worsening confusion. At least a crude estimate of visual and auditory acuity is part of the examination of every old person. Wax in the ears is an easily remedied cause of poor hearing. Other forms of deafness may require a hearing aid. A good deal of patience may be needed to train the elderly person to use an aid properly, especially if poor hearing has been present for some time. The doctor should be on the out-look for flat batteries or dirty battery contacts in hearing aids. For assessment purposes, more powerful amplifiers may be needed and there are several useful portable types. The Seel Easi-Com is widely used by members of our team. The address of the manufacturers is given at the end of the chapter.[9] One of these aids is an important part of the equipment of any psychiatrist working with the elderly. In extremity, a stethoscope used in reverse may help. Visual defects, like hearing defects, vary from those that are easily corrected by spectacles and other aids to those like cataract and glaucoma that require more complicated surgical or medical intervention.

Medication for physical and psychiatric disorders is particularly likely to produce side effects in the elderly and, unless a careful *drug history* is taken, these side effects may be mistaken for a new illness. Antihypertensives, digoxin and diuretics may be responsible for depressive symptoms and all drugs with anti-cholinergic effects (including antidepressants and phenothiazines) may produce confusion and constipation amongst other side effects. Table 2.5 gives a fuller list of drugs that produce confusion. Benzodiazepines often have a 'hangover' effect and may accumulate over many days to produce confusion. Postural hypotension induced by tricyclic antidepressants or phenothiazines may be mistaken for histrionic behaviour and may be dismissed as part of the symptoms of an underlying depressive illness (see Case 4.4). Many drug interactions occur in old people who are more often subject to polypharmacy than the young. When an elderly patient presents with a new symptom, present medication, which may well be causing the symptom, should be reviewed before anything else is added.

Table 2.5: Drugs that have been Reported to Cause or Increase Confusion in Old People

Digoxin	Diuretics
Barbiturates	Indomethacin and other non-steroidal anti-inflammatory drugs
Short- and long-acting benzodiazepines	Septrin
Tricyclic antidepressants	Anti-Parkinsonian drugs
Steriods	
Antihistamines	

Investigations may be planned in the light of findings from the history and examination. There is need for research into the cost-effectiveness of 'screening tests' for potentially reversible dementia. Many doctors would confine themselves to haemoglobin, full blood count and film, urea and electrolytes and thyroid function tests; some would routinely add serum B_{12} and folate and a serological test for syphilis. Other tests such as chest x-ray, skull x-ray, radio-isotope brain scan and computerised axial tomography (CAT) are at present only justified by specific indications. Hopes that CAT might provide an easy and definitive diagnosis of senile dementia by demonstrating brain atrophy have not been realised due to wide overlaps in the picture between normal, functionally ill and demented patients. Nevertheless, research series have shown a small proportion of clinically undetected space-occupying lesions.[10,11,12]

The collection of information is only the first part of the assessment process. Nevertheless, it is vitally important and demands attention to detail and, especially with the elderly, considerable patience. The next chapter goes on to consider the collection of information on family and social circumstances and the principles behind differential diagnosis and the formulation of the patient's problems.

Notes

1. Israel, L., Kozarevic, B. and Sartorius, N., *Source Book of Geriatric Assessment* (S. Karger AG, Basle, 1984).

2. Pattie, A. and Gilleard, C., *Manual of the Clifton Assessment Procedures for the Elderly* (CAPE) (Hodder and Stoughton Educational, Sevenoaks, 1979).

3. Trethowan, W.H. and Sims, A.C.P., *Psychiatry,* (5th edn) (Baillière Tindall, London, 1983).

4. Hodkinson, H.M., 'Evaluation of a Mental Test Score for Assessment of Mental Impariment in the Elderly', *Age and Ageing,* 1, 1972, 223–8.

5. Blessed, G., Tomlinson, B.E. and Roth, M., 'The Association between Quantative Measures of Dementia and Senile Change in the Grey Matter of Elderly People', *British Journal of Psychiatry,* 114, 1968, 797–811.

6. Lishman, W.A., *Organic Psychiatry* (Blackwell Scientific Publications, London, 1978).

7. Cummings, J.L., and Benson, D.F., *Dementia: a Clinical Approach* (Butterworth, Boston, 1983).

8. Caird, F.I. and Judge, T.G., *Assessment of the Elderly Patient* (Pitman Medical Publishing, Tunbridge Wells, 1979).

9. Suppliers of Easi-Com S101: The Seel Company Ltd, 3 Young Square, Livingstone, Scotland.

10. Jacoby, R.J., Levy, R. and Dawson, J.M., 'Computed Tomography in the Elderly: 1 The Normal Population', *British Journal of Psychiatry,* 136, 1980, 249–55.

11. Jacoby, R.J., Levy, R. and Dawson J.M., 'Computed Tomography in the Elderly: 2 Senile Dementia, Diagnosis and functional impairment', *British Journal of Psychiatry,* 136, 1980, 256–69

12. Jacoby, R.J., Levy, R. and Birch, J.M., 'Computed Tomography and the Outcome of Affective Disorder: A Follow-up Study of Elderly Patients', *British Journal of Psychiatry,* 139, 1981, 288–92.

THE CLASSIFICATION OF MENTAL ILLNESS IN OLD AGE, SOCIAL AND FAMILY FACTORS, FORMULATION AND MANAGEMENT PLANS

This book adopts a problem-solving approach rather than one based solely on diagnosis. The chapters on presentations of mental illness in old age are arranged with this in mind. Nevertheless, diagnosis and classification of mental illness are very important if we are to recognise diseases that may respond to specific treatment and in order to test out new methods of treatment. One of the criticisms of much early evaluation of drugs in dementia was that the dementia itself was not identified according to probable aetiology. The doctor who prescribes symtomatically without attention to diagnosis may harm his patients. One of the authors had the misfortune, some years ago, to come across a severely depressed man whose general practitioner had labelled him as 'confused' and who had been prescribed two different laxatives and an anti-diarrhoeal drug. In fact, he was depressed and had faecal retention with overflow incontinence. He responded to appropriate treatment based on appropriate psychiatric and physical diagnosis. There is a risk that the classification of disease, pursued as an end in itself, can lead to the human needs of the patient being ignored. On the other hand, the failure to analyse and classify can lead to inappropriate, unhelpful, and even harmful, treatment.

Classification

The idea that all mental illness in old age is due to senile degeneration is still popular. It is only since the Second World War that the classification of mental disorder in old age has begun to be understood. In 1956 Roth,[1] in a classic research report, described how elderly psychiatric inpatients with different diagnoses had different prognoses measured in simple outcome terms at six months and two years. The measures of outcome he used were: whether the patient was dead, still living in an institution or back at home. The diagnostic categories he looked at in his hospital-based study were: senile psychosis, more recently often referred to as senile dementia Alzheimer's type (SDAT), arteriosclerotic psychosis (multi-infarct dementia, MID), acute confusional states, paraphrenic illnesses and depressive illness. Roth's approach to diagnosis was descriptive. He looked for factors in the mental state and previous history which pointed to a diagnosis and then confirmed the validity of the diagnosis by looking at the natural history of the illness. Medical diagnosis is generally based on such a descriptive approach but additional help is given in classification by the response to different treatments of different disease categories. Ultimately, pathological, biochemical or psycho-social causation, where one or more of these can be established, sets the seal on diagnostic classification. Broadly, there are three different groups of psychiatric diseases corresponding to predominantly structural, biochemical and psycho-social causation. These are enumerated in Figure 3.1.

Any classification represents an over-simplification of reality. In fact, there is considerable overlap. For example, although acute confusional states are classified as organic for descriptive reasons, they are largely caused by acute metabolic upsets associated with physical illness. Affective illness may be associated with anatomoical lesions, for example in stroke illness. The borderline between neurotic and psychotic depressions is not always clear-cut. Nevertheless, Figure 3.1 does give a broadly correct picture. Brief descriptions of the main diagnostic categories follow. Expanded descriptions have been given for conditions not covered in later chapters.

Psychoses

Organic Psychoses

These are the conditions which are usually believed to be based on structural changes in the brain and they affect around 10 per cent of the over-65-year-old population.

Senile Dementia of the Alzheimer Type. (SDAT) This accounts for half of psychiatric hospital inpatients with dementia and is a condition of insidious onset usually presenting first with memory loss and progressing slowly to personality deterioration and the impairment of self-care abilities. The anatomical and biochemical pathology are beginning to be understood but the underlying cause has not been identified although genetic susceptibility has some relevance.

Multi-infarct Dementia. (MID) About 20 per cent of psychiatric hospital patients with dementia suffer from this disease. It is associated with

Figure 3.1: Classification of Mental Illness in Old Age

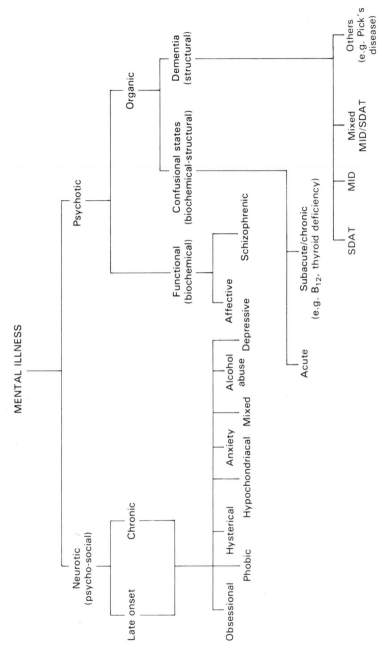

hypertension and stroke illness and often has a relatively sudden onset and stepwise progression. A further fifth of dementias seem to be due to a mixture of SDAT and MID.

Other Dementias. This group includes other dementias of unknown aetiology such as Pick's disease, a group of dementias associated with space-occupying lesions and a group with metabolic causes B_{12} deficiency, thyroid deficiency, etc. which overlap with some of the causes of acute confusional states. The dementias and acute confusional states are discussed in more detail in Chapter 5.

Fuctional Psychoses

These affect 3 to 4 per cent of the over-65-year-old population. They are split into two main groups, with different genetics and aetiology: schizophrenic illness and affective illness.

Schizophrenic Illness. This affects perhaps 1 per cent of the elderly population. Many *chronic schizophrenics* survive into old age. So far the problem of helping these people has been buried in our large mental institutions. As newer generations of schizophrenic patients are cared for in the community, so we can expect that in old age they will need special help. *Late-onset schizophrenia* nearly always takes the form of a paranoid illness ('late paraphrenia') and is discussed in Chapter 7.

Affective Illness. The severe forms of affective illness have a partly genetic and biochemical aetiology although the later the first onset of disease, the less important are the genetic factors. They have been divided into unipolar and bipolar types. Unipolar types have recurrent illness, usually depressive, although a few have recurrent hypomania. Bipolar types have both depressive and hypomanic phases. Recent research has shown that some apparent unipolar depressives have their first attack of hypomania in old age.[2] A possible reason for this is an increased incidence of (non-dementing) brain damage in this population. These illnesses are discussed more fully in Chapter 4.

Neuroses

Neurotic illness affects 12 to 20 per cent of the elderly population.[3,4]. Like other mental illness in old age, it is not detected as often as it should be as people tend to attribute its handicaps to 'old age'. About half of elderly neurotics have had symptoms all their adult lives but another half develop their symptoms for the first time in response to the stresses of late life. Neurosis and personality disorder correspond least well to conventional medical ideas of causation and illness. They are best seen as maladaptive ways of coping with the stresses of life, and although they may have some genetic and biochemical components they are probably chiefly a result of inappropriate learned patterns of behaviour. The commonest form of chronic neurosis is hypochondriacal but new onset or worsening of symptoms may be associated with depressive illness (see Chapter 6). Late-onset neurosis is predominantly of the anxiety-depressive type (although there may also be a mixture of hypochondriachal ideas) and occurs in as many as one-third of physically ill old people. Pure *anxiety-neurosis* is extremely rare in old age. Primary *hysterical neurosis* with histrionic symptoms never occurs in old age. This kind of presentation should lead to the most careful investigation to exclude underlying depressive illness, occult physical illness or organic brain disease. With one exception, *phobic states* rarely present in old age. The exception is the fear of going out, provoked often by postural instability and the fear of fall. It is hard to classify this as 'neurotic' since the fear may be clearly based on physical infirmity. On the other hand, the anxiety component often causes a far greater limitation on activity than the physical one. A new onset of *obsessional neurosis* is also very rare in old age although pre-existing obsessional traits may be emphasised in a depressive illness. *Depressive neurosis* (often with a mixture of other symptoms) is common in old age. Its relationship to depressive illness is a complicated one, and is explored more fully in Chapter 4.

The term *personality disorder* is often used in a perjorative way. If it is used at all in psychiatry, it should refer to abnormal and habitual ways of relating to other people. The use of the term does not absolve the user from trying to understand and help the sufferers. Neither does it mean that the sufferer is immune from psychiatric illness. Indeed, there is often a link between personality type and illness, for example, people with depressive personalities may be more than usually prone to depressive illness. Abnormal personalities are often the result of disturbed relationships in earlier life. Despite such damage, people will often cope well with life provided they are not exposed to abnormal stress. Case 3.1 illustrates these points.

Case 3.1:

 M.S. was a 68-year-old widow. At the age of four her mother died, allegedly as a result of a beating from her husband (although he was never prosecuted). The cause of this beating was that M.S. was an illegitimate child of her mother's lover, conceived while her father was away during the First World War. After her mother's death M.S. was turned out on the street, and taken in by another family. She says they used to go out drinking a lot. At the age of 17 she was hospitalised with TB and on discharge from hospital married a man who flew into unexpected rages, and was later diagnosed as having schizophrenia. She looked after him for many years, but in 1976 he finally went into a hostel. She blamed herself for not looking after him, and had a 'breakdown'. After that, she lived a nomadic life living in boarding houses at various seaside resorts, never very satisfied with her lot, and always anxious and frightened. When seen in 1985, she had returned to her home town, and was about to be ejected from the boarding house in which she was living. She had some mild biological signs of depression and unrealistic expectations that Social Services could immediatedly find her permanent accommodation near her sister. After a further journey to another seaside town, she was admitted for treatment of her depression and assessment of what help could be given for her maladaptive responses to stress. The diagnostic label of 'inadequate personality disorder' could be attached to this lady but although technically correct, it does little justice to the way she coped for years with a schizophrenic husband. After a period of about six months' hospitalisation during which staff refused to reject her, despite awkwardness on her part about finding new accommodation, she was re-housed and will be followed up in the community by a member of our team.

With all these qualifications, some personality patterns can be identified and briefly discussed. *Insecure, rigid* and *anxiety-prone* people have the greatest problems in adapting to old age and seem especially prone to develop depressive symptoms. Paranoid, *isolated* people have a greater risk of developing paranoid illnesses but generally cope well unless physical or psychiatric deterioration leads to the need to accept outside help. Such people will often refuse all help offered and may end up living in extremely squalid and unhealthy circumstances. *Passively dependent* people also cope well as long as they have someone to depend on. They are, however, especially vulnerable to the loss of a spouse or other caring person. *Sociopathic* personalities exercise their abnormal ways of relating within the family or within the institution where they are living. Their anti-social behaviour can make life very difficult for the managers of residential and nursing homes. Disinhibited, anti-social behaviour is also sometimes seen in people with frontal lobe brain damage following chronic heavy drinking, stroke or trauma. Sometimes appropriate psychological approaches can modify this behaviour.

Alcoholism and drug-dependency are largely hidden problems in old age. We still occasionally come across old people who are dependent on barbiturates prescribed for the first time as sleeping tablets many years ago. Old people can become psychologically and physically dependent on benzodiazepine hypnotics. Those atypical elderly depressed patients who are given mono-amine oxidase inhibitors and respond dramatically may become dependent on the mono-amine oxidase inhibitor as when it is withdrawn the depression may return. In this case a kind of dependence may be a reasonable price to pay for a great improvement in the quality of life. As will be apparent from the above, drug dependence in old people is usually related to prescribed drugs and so both its causation and cure are in the hands of doctors.

With a 50 per cent increase in the elderly population and a 100 per cent increase in national alcohol consumption in the UK over the last thirty years, we should expect to see some elderly alcoholics. Nevertheless, the belief persists that alcoholism is rarely, if ever, seen in old age. Studies from as far apart as Scotland,[5] Australia[6] and the USA[7] suggest that the present generation of old people drink less alcohol than their younger contemporaries, but this may be misleading for several reasons. First, owing to differences in average body composition, old people may need less alcohol to become intoxicated[8]. They may also respond differently to survey methods and present figures do not rule out the possibility of a cohort effect as our current generation of heavy drinkers grows older. An epidemiological study in London[9] has shown that for women the prevalence rate for alcoholism continues to rise into the seventh decade whereas for men it peaks in the fifties. Two groups of elderly alcoholics are discernible. Chronic alcoholics who have survived and those, often women, who have turned to alcohol for the first time in response to the stresses of ageing.

Case 3.2:

This 73-year-old widow, living alone, presented initially to the geriatricians with repeated falls. Investigations showed no cause for these falls and she was managed symptomatically. However, about eighteen months after the initial presentation, it became evident that she was abusing alcohol and this was the main cause for her falls. The nephew, who had been bringing her half a bottle of brandy a week, then discovered a cache of empty brandy bottles under the sink and realised that there were different proprietary brands from different sources. The geriatric services alterted the psychiatric services and further psychiatric investigation revealed that she was depressed as a reaction to her rather isolated social circumstances. She had not abused alcohol earlier in life but in response to the stresses she was experiencing, she had started to drink quite heavily which had caused her further problems. She was admitted to the ward in order to correct nutritional deficiencies and enable alcohol-withdrawal under medical cover. The interventions in her social circumstances are discussed later in this chapter.

Often old people with alcohol problems present with falls, self-neglect or unexplained confusion.[10] Their alcohol intake may be concealed by themselves and unknown to, or concealed by, family and friends. Mobility problems sometimes cause them to rely on others for supply. These others may be innocent friends or relatives who are an unwitting part of a large supply network as in Case 3.2 or they may be other alcoholics. If these other alcoholics are close friends or family members, then the prognosis for the old person's alcoholism is worsened. If an old person is admitted to hospital and friends or family members come in drunk, then the possibility that the old person, too, has alcohol problems should be explored. Old people with such problems are especially vulnerable to economic exploitation by other alcoholics, partly because of their frequent dependence on such people for supply of the alcohol and partly because increasing age is a major risk factor for the development of alcoholic dementia with impaired judgement and disinhibition. Late-onset elderly alcoholics with clear social precipitance have relatively good prognosis provided they are willing to accept social change.[11] Chronic alcoholics, especially if they live in an alcoholic culture, are especially difficult to help. A fuller discusion of alcohol abuse in old people by one of the authors is found in the CRC *Handbook of Nutrition in the Aged.*[12]

Social and Family Factors

The elderly person living at home can be conceived of as performing a delicate balancing act (Figure 3.2). The old lady in this illustration balances on a three-legged stool. The legs of her stool are her physical, psychological and social 'health'. The importance of the illustration is that, if any one of the legs is taken away, the old lady tumbles into ill

Figure 3.2: The Balancing Act

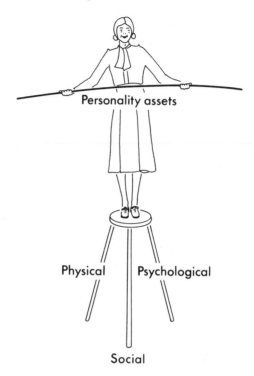

health, and the manner in which this presents may not be related to the underlying cause. Case 3.2 illustrates the point as does the following case.

Case 3.3:

    An elderly widow living alone suddenly became rather breathless.
    Her general practitioner thought that she had had a small myocardial
    infarction and decided to manage her at home. Two days later she
    became acutely disturbed, barricading herself in her room and hurling
    abuse (and small items of furniture) at those who tried to help her.
    The general practitioner made a correct diagnosis of acute confusional
    state secondary to heart failure and myocardial infarction but was
    unable to get her admitted to a general or geriatric hospital because
    of her mental condition. Fortunately, it was possible to admit her to
    a psychiatric unit for the elderly where treatment of her heart failure
    produced a rapid improvement in her mental state.

This is an example of physical illness presenting as a psychiatric crisis. Admission to an acute medical or geriatric unit would have been more appropriate than to a psychiatric hospital; but in this case relatively simple medical management in the psychiatric hospital proved successful. With the continuing improvement in geriatric medical services, this kind of problem need no longer arise.

Analysing Social and Family Matters

The quantitative aspect of social relationships can be summarised neatly by the use of a social network grid.[13] A box is drawn (Figure 3.3). Inside this box the patient's name and age are entered with the names and ages of anyone living in the same household. Down one side of the box, visits to the household by friends and relatives are recorded, with their frequency, and the other side of the box is used in a similar way for statutory helpers. The base of the box can then be used for visits out of the household by the patient.

Figure 3.3: Social Network Diagram of a 73-year-old Alcohol-abusing Widow who presented with Repeated Falls

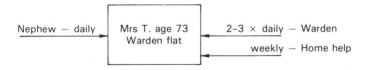

In addition to providing a useful shorthand description of the social network, such a diagram can also be used as the basis for planning social intervention to modify the situation. The interventions used in Case 3.2 are summarised in Figures 3.3 and 3.4. As well as admitting this patient to hospital for treatment, as previously discussed, it was necessary to rearrange her social network (Figure 3.4). With this rearranged social network, her depression showed no signs of returning and the alcohol abuse ceased. Prognosis is not usually so good in elderly patients abusing alcohol and it seems likely that the rearrangement of this lady's social

Figure 3.4: Rearrangement of the Social Network after Inpatient Treatment

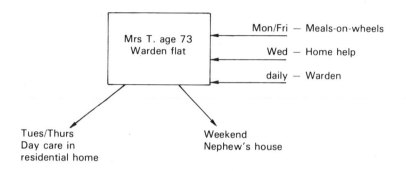

network was the most important factor in preventing a relapse.

The quality of relationships is as important as quantity, but is more difficult to assess objectively. Patterns of relationships can often be detected in the personal history. Family relationships can also be assessed and sometimes modified in joint interviews with the patient and her family. The growing dependence of elderly ill people sometimes puts an extraordinary stress on family relationships. Skill in managing family interviews can only be acquired by practice and is best learned in the presence of an experienced colleague. Traps for the inexperienced include collusion in the pattern of family relationships or ill-timed, unproductive confrontation. Because services are often only made available when a crisis has developed and the family are at the end of their tether, the doctor not uncommonly sees relatives who can be labelled as 'rejecting'. The main answer to this problem lies in the development of effective psychogeriatric, geriatric and social services and the early use of these services by the family. Even when an elderly psychiatrically ill patient does present in a crisis, it may be possible to manage the crisis in such a way that the relatives realise that they can continue to cope with the help of appropriate services.

The most important factor here is a prompt response, usually in the form of a home visit. This is the first step in impressing the family that help is available. The relief of finding someone who has time and is willing to listen to the problems they are facing often helps family members.

The family's assessment of the problems should be taken into account in planning help. The appropriate use of short-term hospital admission, day care and home services to relieve perceived strains can enable families to cope with the difficult problems of a chronically ill elderly relative. Working with the family is considered further in Chapter 8.

When an elderly demented person lives alone, it may be impossible to support her adequately in the community and long-term care in a residential or nursing home or in hospital may be the best solution. Of course, management depends upon the psychiatric diagnosis as well as the family and social factors and it is in understanding the complicated interaction of the various components of the elderly person's situation and finding the best possible management that the skill of the psychogeriatric team resides.

Each person needs a 'tailor-made' plan of medical, psychological and social management. Often it will be necessary to involve members of several different professions in making such a plan. However, the doctor who may be making his initial visit alone, needs to be able to formulate the social and family difficulties and to be able to give a general idea to the family of the help that may be available, including home help, meals-on-wheels, luncheon clubs, day centres, laundry services (sometimes), special apparatus for the disabled and a number of financial allowances, that may be available as a result of legislation. The availability of services varies from area to area but, in the UK, many social service areas are now appointing specialist workers to co-ordinate work with old people and information about services is becoming more widely disseminated.

Problem Formulation and Management

A medical and psycho-social 'diagnosis' is only the beginning of patient management. Not only do many elderly patients have a combination of medical, social and psychological problems, they also frequently have more than one medical or psychiatric diagnosis. Because of this multiplicity of problems, the haphazard management of elderly patients is time-wasting and potentially dangerous. The formulation of the patient's problems as the basis for a management plan that would allow all problems to be tackled simultaneously is crucial. A traditional brief psychiatric formulation such as the example given in Figure 3.5 summarises the patient's living circumstances, the (differential) diagnosis with brief supporting evidence, and any social, personality or other factors important to management, before giving an outline prognosis and management plan. Such a formulation should be supplemented by a carefully-thought-out problem list (Figure 3.6). The aim of this list is to ensure that all points important in the patient's current management are clearly recorded for easy reference. When constructing this list, it is worth bearing in mind the categories of psychological, physical (especially sensory) and social problems. Management plans can then be made for each of the numbered problems in turn, and problems can be checked each time the patient is reviewed to ensure that progress is occuring on all fronts, and that none of the problems is neglected. Without a problem list, workers will often find themselves managing problems sequentially rather than simultaneously. This may result in the patient living at a sub-optimal level at home or being kept in hospital for longer than is really necessary.

Figure 3.5: Brief Psychiatric Formulation

Mr X. is an 82-year-old man who has lived alone in an old terraced house since he was widowed five years ago. He has no close relatives, and neighbours have been alienated because of his past history of heavy drinking, and recent rude refusal of offers of help. For the last two years he has been increasingly confused, disorientated and self-neglectful. He tends to wander out of the house, especially at night. On interview he has moderate memory impairment and disorientation and other signs of cortical brain dysfunction. There is no evidence of functional mental illness, and he is not currently drinking much alcohol. His mother and father are both said to have 'gone senile' in their seventies. The most probable diagnosis is senile dementia, possibly with an alcoholic component. Initial management should be as an inpatient to relieve social tensions and to enable screening for possible treatable causes of dementia. Before he is discharged his home will have to be cleaned up and after discharge close follow-up will be necessary. He is unlikely to make a recovery, but with appropriate supervision he will probably be able to live at home for some years.

Figure 3.6: Problem List

Mr X Age 82 Problem List

1. Mild dementia of uncertain aetiology
2. Alcohol abuse
3. Poor hearing — needs aid
4. Lives alone, will need careful follow-up
5. Self-neglect — dirty house
6. Alienation of neighbours
7. Nocturnal wandering

A further advantage of the problem-orientated approach is that a doctor can assess his own formulation and management plans by comparison with those of his colleagues and also by the outcome in individual patients. Also, problems which consistently cause critical and potentially remediable delays in patient-management (for example, long waiting lists for particular services) can be identified and some attempt made to deal with them. The problem list also serves as a framework for ordering investigations; indeed, some would say that no investigation should be ordered unless the problem on which it might throw light has already been identified.

Conclusion

This chapter has dealt with the classification of mental disease in old age, the need to make an assessment of family and social factors and the formulation of these varied factors in a way that enables a cohesive management plan to be made. The following chapters will deal with some of the main presentations of psychiatric disorder in old people and the last few chapters will discuss psychological and medical treatment.

Notes

1. Roth, M, 'The Natural History of Mental Disorder in Old Age', *Journal of Mental Science,* 101, 1955, 281–301.

2. Shulman, K. and Post, F., 'Bipolar Affective Disorder in Old Age', *British Journal of Psychiatry,* 136, 1980, 26–32.

3. Sims, A.C.P., *Neurosis in Society* (Macmillan, London, 1983).

4. Bergmann, K. 'Neurosis in Old Age', in T. Arie (ed.), *Health Care of the Elderly', (Croom Helm, London, 1981).*

5. Dight, S., *Scottish Drinking Habits: a Survey of Scottish Drinking Habits and Attitudes to Alcohol* (Office of Population Censuses and Surveys, Her Majesty's Stationery Office, London, 1976).

6. Encel, S. Kotowicz, K.C. and Resler, H.E., 'Drinking Patterns in Sydney, Australia', *Quarterly Journal of Studies on Alcoholism Supplement,* 6, 1972

7. Cahalan, D., Cisin, I.M. and Crossley, H.M., *American Drinking Practices — A National Study of Drinking Behaviour and Attitudes,* (Monographs of the Rutgers Center of Alcohol Studies, No. 6, New Brunswick, New Jersey, 1969).

8. Vestal, R.E., McGuire, E.A., Tobin, J.D., Andres, R., Norris, A.H. and Mezey, E., 'Ageing and Ethanol Metabolism', *Clinical Pharmacology and Therapeutics,* 21, 1977, 3, 343–54.

9. Edwards, G., Hanker, A., Hensman, C., Peto, J. and Williamson, V., 'Alcoholics Known or Unknown to Agencies: Epidemiological Studies in a London Suburb', *British Journal of Psychiatry,* 123, 1973, 169–83.

10. Wattis, J.P., 'Alcohol Problems in the Elderly', *Journal of the American Geriatrics*

Society, XXIX, 1981, 3, 131.

11. Rosin, A.J. and Glatt, M.M., 'Alcohol Excess in the Elderly', *Quarterly Journal of Studies in Alcoholism*, 32, 1971, 53–9.

12. Wattis, J., 'Alcohol and Psychiatric Problems' in R.R. Watson (ed.), *Handbook of Nutrition in the Aged* (CRC Press, Boca Raton, Florida, 1985).

13. Capildeo, R., Court, C. and Rose, F.C., 'Social Network Diagram', *British Medical Journal*, 1976, 1, 143–4.

4 DEPRESSION

The feeling of depression is something we have all experienced. The 'Monday morning' feeling is familiar to most of us. When feelings of depression, often mixed with anxiety, pervade our lives, then there is something wrong that may be helped medically or psychologically. Because depression is a more or less universal experience, the dividing line between normal experience and the milder forms of 'depressive illness' is difficult and so figures for prevalence of these forms of depression vary widely. On the other hand, the more severe forms have relatively clear symptomatology and are easier to detect reliably.

Classification

Psychiatrists vary in how they classify different types of depression and how they relate one type of depression to others.[1] The main argument is as to whether depression is best regarded as a wide spectrum of disorder varying from the mild to the severe or whether it is best seen as two separate conditions (perhaps with some overlap) but of essentially different cause. These two different models are illustrated in Figure 4.1, along with the main diagnostic terms used. The mild/severe classification is descriptive but with some aetiological implications and the 'reactive/endogenous' classification makes strong aetiological assumptions. For practical purposes, these arguments seem rather sterile. A description of the patient's condition and an estimation of the relative importance of early learning, current psycho-social stress, genetic endowment and biochemical features seems of more practical use in our present state of knowledge. The question should not be whether a person's depression should be treated biochemically, psychologically or socially but what mixture of these approaches is appropriate to the individual. The following description of categories has been found useful by the authors. A more formal and complete classfication can be found in the diagnostic and statistical manual of the American Psychiatric Association (DSM III)[2] or the glossary to the World Health Organisation's International Classification of Diseases (ICD 9).[3]

'Depressive neurosis' is used to describe people whose habitual outlook in response to life is depressed. There is often an admixture of

51

Figure 4.1: Models of Depression and Diagnostic Terms

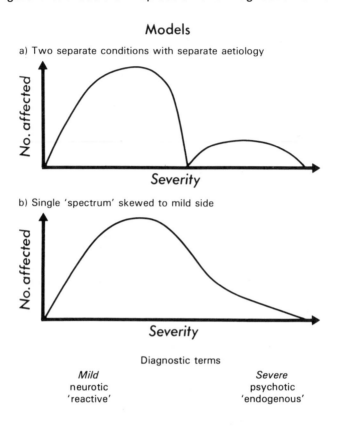

Models

a) Two separate conditions with separate aetiology

b) Single 'spectrum' skewed to mild side

Diagnostic terms

Mild	*Severe*
neurotic	psychotic
'reactive'	'endogenous'

anxiety. Theoretically, the roots of this kind of problem are based in life experience rather than in genetically determined biochemical change. As far as old people are concerned, they may have had this problem all their lives or they may have started to behave this way for the first time in response to the stresses of late life.

'Depressive psychosis' ('endogenous depression', 'manic depressive psychosis — depressed type') implies that depression is so severe that the person is out of touch with reality. Aetiologically, this diagnosis suggests that there are biochemical changes and an important genetic contribution although it is recognised that the latter is less important in late-onset severe depression. At the severest end of the spectrum, the sufferers may neglect basic needs and have delusions that they are dead or that their bodies or bowels are rotting away ('nihilistic delusions').

When people are so depressed, they may become mute and unresponsive to their environment ('depressive stupor'). A slightly less severe clinical picture presents with delusions with depressive content (guilt, unworthiness, poverty, ill health) or sometimes with paranoid, persecutory content. As the patient lapses into or recovers from such a state, they may go through a period of increased anxiety, sometimes with profoundly histrionic behaviour such as undressing in public or constantly demanding attention and reassurance. There can be great clinical similarity to the picture of 'neurotic depression'. Depression often emphasises the worst aspects of personality and helpers have to beware of the trap of relatives who say 'she's always been like this' when they really mean she has always had these tendencies to, for example, excessive dependency, but these have got worse recently. For a full research-based description of depressive illness in old people see Post.[4]

'Reactive depression' is a term which has been used as synonymous with 'depressive neurosis' or to define a group of depressions which are a reaction to life circumstances and recover spontaneously when these improve. In old age, severe depressive illness is not infrequently a reaction to bereavement, and may require a medical as well as psychological treatment before it resolves. 'Reactivity of mood' has also been used to describe the capability of some less severely depressed patients to 'cheer up' when in company, meeting the grandchildren, etc. Because of its varied usage, reactive depression should be avoided as a diagnostic term although it is still perfectly legitimate to use it descriptively. *'Pervasive depression'* is a concept which has been used by epidemiologists to describe depression of a severity or type likely to warrant and respond to medical or psychological intervention. It would include all those we have grouped under 'depressive psychosis' and a proportion of those who might be labelled 'depressive neurosis'.

Prevalence

Epidemiological studies are notoriously difficult to conduct in psychiatry, especially when the elderly age group is included.[5] Depressive disorders as diagnosed by psychiatrists peak in mid-life. Milder ('neurotic') depressions peak before 40 years of age, more severe disorders later. Women outnumber men in all depressive diagnoses earlier in life but by the age of 65 years, the prevalence is more or less equal. A fair estimate of overall prevalence rates over 65 is about 2 to 3 per cent for severe 'psychotic' depressions and 14 per cent or more for

Figure 4.2: Phases of Biochemical Vulnerability to Depression

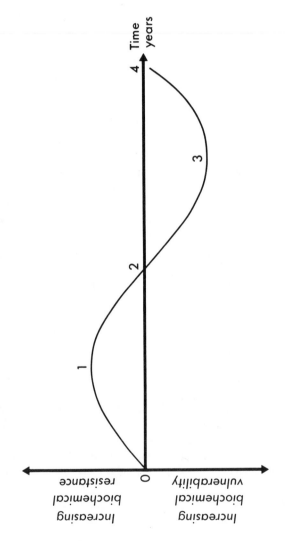

'pervasive depressions'. Studies which have looked for *symptoms* associated with depression rather than a psychiatric diagnosis show a progressive increase of symptoms with increasing age in the over-20-year-old adult. When depressive symptoms have been used as screening criteria to identify patients who may be suffering from pervasive depression, as many as 40 per cent of the elderly have been found to have these symptoms. Several explanations for this are possible. One might be that transitory depressive phenomena which would not satisfy research diagnostic criteria for depressive illness are commoner in old age. Another might be that psychiatrists are more reluctant to make a diagnosis of depressive disorder with increasing age and yet another that certain physical signs and symptoms in old age might be mistakenly seen as signs of depression.

Aetiology

Genetic Susceptibility and Life Events

The inheritance of a tendency towards severe depressive illness and hypomania is well documented. With late-onset illness, genetic factors are generally less important than for earlier-onset cases. A link between the onset of severe depression in old age and major life events such as bereavement has been clearly demonstrated.[6] One theory that has been put forward to explain why people with an inherited tendency develop depressive illness in response to some stresses and not in response to others is that the predisposition is expressed in phasic periods of biochemical vulnerability (Figure 4.2).

Quite a severe life even might be weathered at point 1, a fairly major trauma might be needed to initiate a depressive attack at point 2 but at point 3 a minor trauma might suffice. This model also explains why antidepressant therapy often has to be continued for months but can then usually be withdrawn without a recurrence of depression, at least in the short term. Between points 2 and 4 in the figure, once the depressive illness had started, biochemical treatment might be needed to suppress the symptoms. Once point 4 is reached, the treatment is no longer needed. This model would allow for different periodicity in different sufferers and for biochemically mediated increasing frequency of vulnerable periods with increasing age. Although theoretically attractive, it is not easy to prove or disprove this model experimentally.

Biochemical Theories

Various brain amines, notably noradrenaline (NA) and 5-hydroxytriptamine (5HT, serotonin) and their metabolic products have been found to be depleted in the brains of patients who have died whilst severely depressed. Studies on urine and cerebo-spinal fluid have also shown decreased metabolites of these neurotransmitters although there has been much argument about the significance of these findings. The interaction of different neurotransmitter systems has resulted in debate as to whether the primary deficiency is of noradrenaline or 5-hydroxytriptamine. A deficiency of dopamine (DA), another brain amine, is associated with Parkinson's disease, relatively common in old age and very frequently associated with depressed mood. Drugs which decrease brain amines (e.g. reserpine) have been shown to produce depression and at least some of the drugs used to treat depression may work by enhancing the availability of amines at brain receptor sites. Interesting biochemical findings in normal ageing are small decreases in brain amines and an increase in blood platelet mono-amine oxidasive activity. Mono-amine oxidases are concerned with the breakdown of transmitters such as NA and 5HT. These changes superimposed on the phases of vulnerability already postulated in Figure 4.2 might explain the clinically observed tendency to increasing frequency of depression as people with recurrent depressive illness grow older. The effect of biochemical ageing could be to shift the horizontal axis on this model upwards, thus increasing the vulnerable periods.

A subgroup of elderly depressed patients has been found in neurophysiological[7] and computerised axial tomography (CAT scan)[8,9] studies who have findings mid-way between those of normal controls and demented patients. They do not generally go on to develop dementia but they may represent a subgroup of elderly depressed patents who have a structural cause for their depression. In this context, it is interesting, too, that depression following stroke is significantly related to the location of the lesion on CAT scan.[10]

Bereavement

Following bereavement, four stages of normal grieving have been described in our society.[11] An initial stage of numbness is followed by a period of restlessness and pining. A time of anger comes next, sometimes directed at helping professionals, sometimes at the deceased or sometimes inwardly with accompanying guilt. During this phase, mild depression of mood is normal but sometimes the depression may go 'out of control' and the sufferer then exhibits all the features of severe depressive illness, including a particularly high risk of suicide. This is not the only cause of increased death in bereaved people. In men especially, the death rate from physical illness in the year following bereavement increases beyond chance expectation and three-quarters of these deaths are due to heart problems. People really do seem to die of a 'broken heart'. Somatic anxiety symptoms, headache and digestive upsets, are other common concomitants of bereavement. The final phase of normal grieving is a resolution and adaptation to life without the dead person. The process of grieving is individual and to a large extent culturally determined.[12] The phases described above can merge one with another, and need not be in the order described. The recently bereaved are a 'high-risk' group who merit special attention from health service professionals to enable them, if necessary, to work through their feelings of depression and bereavement and to enable the professionals to detect and treat early any depression which seems to be getting out of control. We have come across a group of elderly depressed bereaved people (mostly women) who find it very hard to talk about, or show much apparent emotion concerning, their lost spouse. Persistent bereavement work may be necessary to unlock this stubborn kind of grief, perhaps in a day hospital setting.

Social Factors

Recent research has shown that severe life events such as bereavement, major social difficulties and poor health act as provoking factors for depressive illness in old people. Old people without a close, confiding relationship were rendered especially vulnerable to the operation of such provoking factors.[6]

Psychological Theories

A psychological model of depression has been evolved by Seligman[13]. He has shown, through animal experiments, that where outcome is made independent of behavioural response, animals lapse into a state of 'learned helplessness' which, he argues, is in many ways analogous to the human experience of depressive illness. He has also demonstrated depletion of noradrenaline in the brains of experimental animals, thus providing a link between psychological and biochemical theories. The learned helplessness is very difficult to remove once it has been induced although, if the animal is repeatedly shown that its response does now make some difference, it may gradually recover. The relevance to old people is that they, too, are subject to unpleasant events, over which they have little apparent control. Compulsory retirement is usual, however good someone is at their job and however much they may wish to continue. Physical disabilities may accumulate despite efforts to keep fit. This theory would, therefore, be one explanation of the remarkable association of depression with physical illness in old age. Old friends may seem to die off at an alarming rate providing a link between the learned-helplessness theory, bereavement and depression. Seligman's theory, although it has been useful in reinforcing the idea that the facilitation of the elderly person's sense of control is an important task for any service provision, has not proved as helpful in generating practical ideas as to how to intervene with the elderly depressed individual.

In contrast, Beck[14] developed a cognitive theory of depression which gives a detailed description of a therapeutic approach and procedures which could be used with somebody who is depressed. Cognitive therapy emphasises the role of the individual's evaluation of any situation in determining both mood and behaviour (see Figure 8.2). The more an individual inaccurately evaluates any life situation in a negative way, the greater the risk of becoming depressed. Therapeutic interventions are aimed at improving the individual's abiliity to evaluate accurately their life experiences, and thus change their behaviour and reduce depressed affect (see Case 6.3). Although interventions using a cognitive approach may need adaptation to take account of the special needs of the elderly arising from ageing (see Chapter 8), Beck has provided us with an important extra 'tool' which can be used with depressed elderly people either in groups or on an individual basis. Indeed, of all psychotherapeutic approaches to depression, cognitive therapy has the most empirical evidence supporting its efficacy.

Prognosis

Recent findings have suggested that of depressed patients who present to the hospital service, just over one-third have a good outcome at one year, a similar proportion deteriorate or die and a smaller fraction remain unchanged.[15] The association with physical illness and uncontrollable life events such as bereavement and admission to an institution suggest possible mediators for this poor prognosis. Other factors associated with a poor prognosis are duration of more than one or two years before treatment, increasing age, and severity (see Table 4.1). We believe that a 'whole person' approach to depressed elderly patients can improve prognosis. We can look at some of the prognostic factors in Table 4.1 in this light. Increased duration of depression may mean that, in addition to biochemical changes, the patient has also developed depressive 'habits' and that the family and neighbours have evolved compensatory ways of behaving. These habits and compensatory behaviours tend to perpetuate the depressive behaviour, even when the underlying biochemical abnormality is corrected. The patient who has been depressed for a long time, therefore, demands not only appropriate biochemical treatment but also a careful psychological evaluation of living circumstances and modification of depressive 'habits'. Severity of depression may be a prognostic factor because people with very severe depression are sometimes treated inadequately. The popular pressure against ECT and the inconveniences in the UK of getting a second opinion, not just from a local expert doctor, but under the 1983 Mental Health Act from a remote 'mental health commissioner', may deter doctors from using this effective treatment. In some states of the USA and some European countries, the campaign against the abuse of ECT has resulted in it becoming unavailable to those that need it. Severely depressed patients are notoriously poor in their compliance with medication and so when patients are discharged home before they are completely 'well', it is very easy for them to stop taking tablets and for relapse to occur. Careful follow-up can help here. Associated physical illness may need active treatment and review. We clearly cannot prevent a traumatic life event, such as bereavement, for patients who have been depressed, but we can ensure that there is somebody, either friend of professional, who is available to support them through such life events. Poor physical design in psychiatric units can reduce the chances of successful treatment by reducing self-esteem, opportunities for interpersonal interactions and mobility. Staff skills and attitudes are also relevant here. This is discussed further in Chapter 9. Thus, at least some of the factors associated with poor prognosis may be amenable to careful intervention. Case 4.1 is a good example of how a 'poor prognosis' can be turned into a happy life with this approach.

Case 4.1:

Mrs B.R. was a 60-year-old married lady with a history of chronic depression. She had been admitted to the psychiatric unit 16 times

Table 4.1: Factors Associated with Poor Prognosis in Depressed Old People

Psychotic illness with depressive delusions
Increased duration of illness
Physical illness
Low social class (more likely to suffer severe life events)
housing difficulties
low income
Severe life events in the year after the initial episode

Source: Based on Murphy, (1985)[15]

in 14 years and had never been well for any sustained period since the age of 55 years when her mother died. After her first admission under our care she was discharged home but refused to come to day hospital and took to her bed. She had nihilistic delusions (that she had no pulse) and was readmitted. When her previous history was thoroughly reviewed it was evident that she had always failed to take adequate doses of antidepressants because of alleged side effects. She also behaved in a highly dependent way and her relationship with her husband was one of mutual hostility. She was put on a compulsory treatment section of the Mental Health Act and treated using gradually increasing doses of tricyclic antidepressant. Despite an observed improvement in her mood over several months, she maintained she felt no better and hostile-dependent behaviour continued. A behavioural cognitive treatment programme was instituted and slow improvement continued. She and her husband seemed unable to appreciate this and an extremely hostile interaction continued. Marital therapy was instituted and after six months in hospital the point was reached where she could be discharged. Despite her attendance at day hospital while on the ward, on discharge she refused to attend further, and weekly home visits were carried out by the psychologist and a member of the ward staff. At first, the situation at home caused concern, as she took to lying in bed until lunchtime, complaining of pain. However, the nursing assistant noticed on one visit that Mrs B.R. was showing signs of arthritis in her hands (not apparent on the ward). This was treated, and she continued to improve slowly. The final 'intervention', a housing transfer, which had been given medical priority, enabled her to live near one daughter and her grandchildren. This allowed her to have a meaningful and constructive family life again, and was agreed with the daughter (both the daughters had been closely involved throughout treatment). Over the months, therapeutic support was gradually reduced, the daughters continuing to slowly 'rehabilitate' their mother, and two years later, she remains extremely well, despite having discontinued her antidepressant medication a year ago.

This case illustrates how even severely and chronically depressed old people can be helped with a sustained and co-ordinated approach to treatment. If any of the interventions (medical, psychological and social) had been mistimed, inappropriately carried out, or missed completely, this old person might have continued to relapse and to live an unhappy and unfulfilled life.

Management

Assessment

The proper assessment of a depressed old person involves much more than just making a diagnosis. Figure 4.3 summarises the interactive model of depression outlined in this chapter. Periodic phases of vulnerability to depression, genetically determined and biochemically mediated, are the basis of severe recurrent depressive illness. However, a severe depressive illness can also arise *de novo* in old age in response to a major stress such as bereavement and may have the same 'biological' features (e.g. early morning wakening and diurnal variation of mood) that we associate with recurrent depressive illness. People who have evolved maladaptive styles of coping with life at an early age, especially those who are rigid, insecure or over-anxious, may be more susceptible not only to neurotic but also to psychotic depression in old age. All depressions may be complicated by depressive 'habits' of behaviour and the way that other people in the environment react to these. Assessment is not, therefore, a question of just deciding whether this depression is 'psychotic' or 'neurotic' but of determining the balance of initiating and maintaining causes from the selection in Figure 4.3.

Figure 4.3: Factors Contributing to Causing and Maintaining Depression

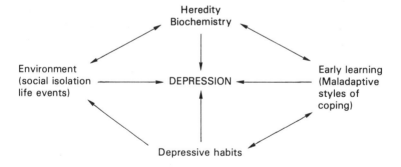

History

This should be obtained from an independent informant as well as from the patient. The time course of the illness should be ascertained as well as its severity and how far it is threatening life by self-neglect or suicidal intent. The patient's previous personality and any previous episodes of affective illness should be investigated. A family history of affective illness or suicide should be sought. Possible precipitating factors in the environment (e.g. bereavement, ill health and other 'loss events') should be explored. A special note should be made of any alteration in behaviour of friends and relatives in response to the patient's illness as this may have to be dealt with as part of the patient's treatment.

Mental State

The patient's cleanliness and general appearance and behaviour should be noted. If she lives alone, a tour of the house may reveal an empty larder and other signs of recent self-neglect. One depressed old lady had the previous few weeks' meals-on-wheels deliveries stacked in a cupboard! The patient will often appear depressed but sometimes all her energy will be invested in hypochondriacal or persecutory complaints and she may then not admit to *feeling* depressed. Sleep disturbance, especially early morning wakening and diurnal variation of mood (usually feeling worse in the morning), are characteristic of the more severe depressions. Loss of the ability to take pleasure in anything and loss of drive are other common findings. Thoughts are often preoccupied with ideas of poverty, guilt or illness and these worries may reach delusional intensity. The speed of thought and talk may be profoundly slowed. This depressive retardation may co-exist with agitation, a very uncomfortable state of affairs for the patient. Retardation is also one of the factors that can produce apparent cognitive impairment. If given plenty of time, the retarded patient may improve his performance on cognitive tests.

Psychomotor slowing is also a feature of the 'subcortical' syndrome (see Chapter 5) and its presence should always lead to consideration of special investigations such as tests for vitamin B_{12} and thyroid deficiency. In difficult cases, perhaps the best test of whether cognitive impairment is secondary to depression is to treat the depression and see if cognitive function and behaviour improve. It should also never be forgotten that dementia confers no immunity to depression and indeed multi-infarct dementia often leads to depressed mood. In these cases, cautious use of antidepressant treatment is fully justified.

Physical Examination

Depressed mood is associated with physical illness in old age. Stroke illness, especially with lesions in the frontal or occipito-parietal regions, is often associated with the depressed mood.[10] Depression may be the first presentation of a hidden neoplasm. There are particularly strong relationships between depression and cardiovascular disease and depression and Parkinsonism. Metabolic upsets, especially electrolyte imbalance, thyroid deficiency and vitamin B_{12} deficiency, are associated with depression in old age. A physical examination and appropriate biochemical and haematological investigation are, therefore, mandatory.

Problem Formulation

Having assembled the data, it is essential to formulate the problems and prepare a management plan. All factors should be taken into account and a problem list is an effective way of doing this. A particularly important decision is whether the patient should be initially treated at home or in hospital and social circumstances as well as severity of illness and suicide risk are important in this decision. The following case-histories illustrate some of the important points in management of depression. More details of physical and psychological treatments for depression are given in Chapters 8 to 10.

Case 4.2:

A 72-year-old married women had a history of two previous attacks of a severe depresssive illness, the last only in the previous year. She lost interest in her husband and house over a period of a few weeks and became extremely agitated. Her relatives were distressed and feared she might take an overdose. The general practitioner was called in and the psychiatrist was consulted. The old lady confided in him that, as a result of liason with a soldier during the war, she believed that she had contracted venereal disease and this was allegedly ruining her husband and daughter (both perfectly healthy people). This depressive delusion was held in the face of all evidence to the contrary.

Eventually she was persuaded to accept inpatient treatment with ECT, although she was convinced it would not do any good. She made a full recovery and has remained well on lithium therapy. Her depression was almost entirely of the 'biological' type and presented in a straightforward way, which is relatively unusual in elderly people.

Case 4.3:

This 82-year-old lady was gradually losing her sight. She was of German extraction and had successfully coped with the Second World War and its aftermath, despite living in the Communist-occupied zone. She had subsequently escaped to England with her husband, where she enjoyed an active life, bringing up her family and teaching German and continental cookery. She found the restrictions of old age, especially her deteriorating eyesight, extremely difficult to cope with and began to respond by spending a lot of time in bed. She took a small overdose of nitrazepam and the general practitioner referred her for a psychiatric opinion.

She had none of the biological features of severe depression, although her mother had, in fact, committed suicide following the Second World War. The diagnosis was of a late-onset depressive neurosis reactive to her deteriorating eyesight and restricted lifestyle. With some trepidation the decision was made to treat her at home with twelve weekly sessions of 'cognitive' psychotherapy. She made an excellent response, despite some early problems, gradually resuming previous activities and learning to cope with her poor eyesight. She has now had an operation for her cataract and is looking forward to the increased independence her improved eyesight will bring.

Case 4.4:
A widow in her seventies became depressed when her daughter's marriage broke up and the daughter and grand-daughter moved into her small flat. She could not cope and went to her general practitioner, who prescribed imipramine. Unfortunately, she was already receiving a beta-blocking drug and she developed severe postural hypotension which necessitated hospital admission. Once the daughter and grand-daughter were found alternative accommodation nearby, her depression lifted and she did not need drugs.

These case-histories illustrate the variety of different presentations of depression in old age and the variety of approaches needed to cope with them. A true multidisciplinary approach offers the best hope for the old person. Figure 4.4 is a flow chart intended to aid the *diagnosis* of depression in old age. It should not be used by itself to plan management. The idea that psychotic depressions only ever require physical treatment (drugs, ECT) and neurotic depressions only ever require psychological treatments is based on a falsely dichotomous view of human nature as Case 4.1 well illustrates. Many depressed patients will require a mixture of physical treatment and psychological and social help if they are to be given the best chance of recovery. The proportion of these different ingredients to the management plan will, of course, vary from patient to patient as Cases 4.1 to 4.4 demonstrate. The timing of interventions is also crucial. Thus, a woman with marital problems and delusional depression might require inpatient therapy with ECT followed by marital therapy. To put the marital therapy first could waste time in unsuccessful efforts with the patient not in a state to respond. To ignore

Figure 4.4: Flow Chart of the Diagnosis of a Patient with Depressed Mood

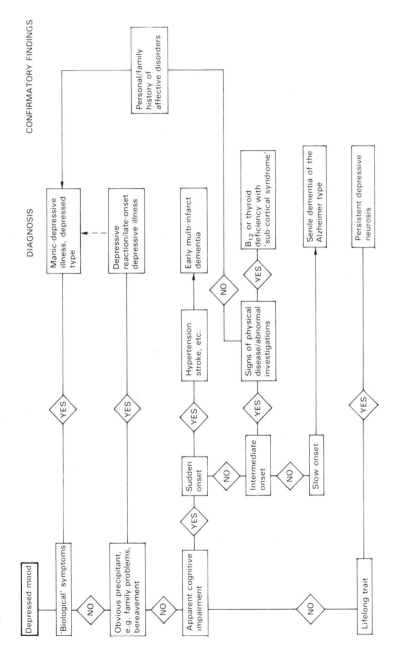

the marital problem after ECT might be to make full recovery less likely and relapse more probable. Management should be planned as a problem-solving exercise with the problems arranged according to the order in which they should be tackled.

Prevention

Improving family relationships and the capacity to make meaningful choices in later life would presumably protect some old people against depression as would the prompt diagnosis and effective treatment of physical illness. Counselling for the chronically sick about the nature of their illness and ways to overcome disability might also help. Extra support and, if necessary, formal counselling for the recently bereaved might avoid some depressive illness in this group. It might also help to reduce the excessive mortality from physical, especially cardiovascular, problems. The routine prescription of tricyclic antidepressants to bereaved people should be avoided as it may increase the risk of cardiovascular deaths and, as with the use of tranquillisers, interfere with normal griev-ing. Once depression has occurred, sustained physcial treatment with antidepressants and/or lithium may be needed to prevent recurrence. Psychotherapeutic approaches (e.g. cognitive therapy) may be needed to improve the person's self-image and problem-solving ability. Day hospital or day centre support can help the lonely and, if threatening life events occur, prompt intervention can reduce the risk of repeated depression. Family therapy can help re-establish a healthy role for the sufferer in home life. These are all common-sense approaches. It is diffi-cult to verify their effectiveness experimentally (except for drug maintenance therapy) but case-studies do suggest that these are effec-tive and worthwhile interventions especially in preventing recurrence of depression.

Hypomania

This is much less common than depression in late life and is very rarely seen except in the context of previous episodes of affective disorder. A fair proportion of people with recurrent depressive illness develop hypomania for the first time in late life and a significant number have organic brain damage (not dementia).[16] Over-activity without cognitive impariment is the cardinal clinical feature. The elation and infectious good humour of the younger hypomanic may be replaced by irritability and querulousness. Grandiose ideas and delusions are entertained sometimes with a mixture of paranoid, persecutory ideas. Alcohol abuse with frontal lobe impairment may mimic hypomania although excessive drinking may also sometimes be symptomatic of hypomania. The association between alcoholic brain damage and late-onset hypomania is not clear. There is usually no cognitive impairment though this may have to be inferred indirectly as the patient will not always co-operate with detailed mental state examination. Mixed-mood states with hypomanic over-activity but depressive ideas also occur. The patient is often extremely difficult to help and inpatient treatment, often under a compulsory order, is usually necessary. Response to initial treatment with neuroleptics is usually good. Lithium can also be used in the acute phase. If the affective illness is recurrent, with more than one episode per year, then continuing lithium therapy is appropriate. The use of lithium in old people demands careful monitoring because of risks of toxicity but the excellent results fully justify the risk. Environmental and family factors, especially those likely to lead to poor compliance such as living alone, must be taken into account. A patient who has been chronically hypomanic needs an extended period of stability in hospital and particularly careful rehabilitation if relapse is to be avoided.

Notes

1. Kendell, R.E., 'The Classification of Depression: A Review of Contemporary Confusion', *British Journal of Psychiatry*, 129, 1976, 15–28

2. American Psychiatric Association Task Force on Nomenclature and Statistics, *Diagnostic and Statistical Manual of Mental Disorders*, 3rd ed (American Psychiatric Association, Washington DC, 1980).

3. World Health Organisation, *International Classification of Diseases, Ninth Revision, Mental Disorders, Glossary and Guide*, (Geneva, 1978).

4. Post, F., 'Functional Disorders', in K. Levy and F. Post (eds), *The Psychiatry of Late Life*, (Blackwell Scientific Publications, London, 1982).

5. Gurland, B.J., 'The Comparative Frequency of Depression in Various Age Groups', *Journal of Gerontology*, 31, 1976, 3, 283–92.

6. Murphy, E. 'Social Origins of Depression in Old Age', *British Journal of Psychiatry*, 141, 1982, 135–42.

7. Hendrickson, E. Levy, R. and Post, F., 'Averaged Evoked Responses in Relation to the Cognitive and Affective State of Elderly Patients', *British Journal of Psychiatry*, 134, 1979, 494–500.

8. Jacoby, R., Levy, R. and Bird, J.M. 'Computed Tomography and the Outcome of Affective Disorder: A Follow-up Study of Elderly Patients, *British Journal of Psychiatry*, 139, 1981, 288–92.

9. Jacoby, R., Dolan, R. Levy, R. and Baldy, R., 'Quantative Computed Tomography in Elderly Depressed Patients, *British Journal of Psychiatry*, 143, 1983, 124–7.

10. Lipsey, J.R., Robinson, R.G., Pearlson, G.D., Rao, K. and Price, T.R., 'Mood Change following Bilateral Hemisphere Brain Injury', *British Journal of Psychiatry*, 143, 1983, 266–73.

11. Parkes, C.M., *Bereavement: Studies of Grief in Adult Life*, (Pelican, London, 1976).

12. Parkes, C.M., 'Bereavement', *British Journal of Psychiatry*, 146, 1985, 11–17.

13. Seligman, M.E.P., *Helplessness: On Depression, Development and Death*, (Freeman, San Francisco, 1975).

14. Beck, A.T., Rush, A.S., Shaw, B.E. and Emery, G., *Cognitive Therapy of Depression* (Guilford Press, New York, 1979).

15. Murphy, E. 'The Prognosis of Depression in Old Age', *British Journal of Psychiatry*, 142, 1983, 111–19.

16. Shulman, K. and Post, F. 'Bipolar Affective Disorder in Old Age', *British Journal of Psychiatry*, 136, 1980, 26–32.

5 CONFUSION

It is almost axiomatic that the confused patient does not ask for medical or social help. The general practitioner or social services are called in by worried relatives or neighbours or the confusion is noticed when the patient is admitted to hospital for some other reason. Helping the confused patient is a difficult task for a variety of reasons. The doctor or social worker may lack the proper background knowledge and skills to understand the causes of the patient's confusion; the community support and instititutional care services are generally grossly inadequate and often the patient is not particularly co-operative in using those services which are available.

Demography and Social Policy

This chapter deals with both transient acute confusional states and the more chronic states generally called the dementias. Because acute confusional states are transient and because they are often associated with severe physical illness, their exact prevalence is hard to measure and they are excluded from this section on demography and social policy. The demography of the dementias has already been briefly discussed in Chapter 1. The overall prevalence rate for dementia in the over-65s is around 10 per cent rising from 2 or 3 per cent of the 65-69-year age group to over 20 per cent of over-80-year-old people.[1] Not only do this group have more physical and social handicaps, they are also more likely to need continuing institutional care. Further, senile dementia in the very elderly seems to be a less rapidly fatal condition and overall survival of the elderly demented has increased over the last twenty-five years or so.[2] The implication of this and of the decreasing ratio of middle-aged to elderly people is that more community care and more institutional care will be needed over the next twenty years. This has been pointed out repeatedly. In 1981 the Office of Health Economics produced a report on dementia in old age,[1] the *British Medical Journal* has carried several leaders on this subject, one of them aptly titled 'Dementia, The Quiet Epidemic',[3] and the Health Advisory Service, a body charged with ensuring adequate care for disadvantaged elderly people in the health and social services, produced in 1982 a report entitled

'The Rising Tide'[4] dealing in detail with some of the implications of these changes. Despite this, government response has been woefully inadequate. Attempts have been made to shift some of the burden away from the health and social services on to private enterprise but these have been based on political dogma rather than any certainty that this is a better or even a cheaper way of caring. In the authors' opinion, the way in which we treat our old people now, especially those suffering from dementia, will be regarded in the future in much the same way as we regard the slave-trade in the eighteenth century or child-labour in the nineteenth century. It will be a major social scandal and a blemish on the face of our 'affluent society'.

Euthanasia

After visiting some old people's homes or long stay wards for demented patients, colleagues sometimes ask whether euthanasia would not be a better solution, especially in view of the poor 'quality of life' of the old people. Quite apart from the moral question of whether we have the right to terminate our own or anybody else's life, the practical question of why quality of life is poor has to be examined. Demented people are far more dependent on the environment in which they live than young people or than well old people. When nurse-staffing levels are often at a quarter or a half of recommended levels, when occupational therapy services on the wards are virtually non-existent and when the wards themselves are often badly designed relics in remote Victorian asylums, it is not surprising if quality of life is not all that good. The shift to well-staffed, well-designed units located in the local community is expensive and is therefore often repeatedly delayed as more glamorous areas of health service expenditure continue to expand. The planning process within the health service has, until recently, allowed uncontrollable growth in many areas of expenditure whilst plans for improving care for old people have continually been put off. It is easy to demonstrate how disability levels measured on scales such as the modified Crichton Royal or the Clifton Behavioural scale (see Chapters 2 and 9) can improve when an individual patient is moved from a poorly staffed ward or old people's home to a well-staffed one. The danger of the euthanasia argument is that it is cheaper to allow old people to die when they need not than to provide adequate community services or institutional care. We are in danger of falling into the same trap as our ancestors by regarding old people as less than human in much the same way that they regarded slaves as disposable personal property. In the following sections we intend to demonstrate that not all confusion in old people is due to

Figure 5.1: Time Course of Different Causes of Confusion

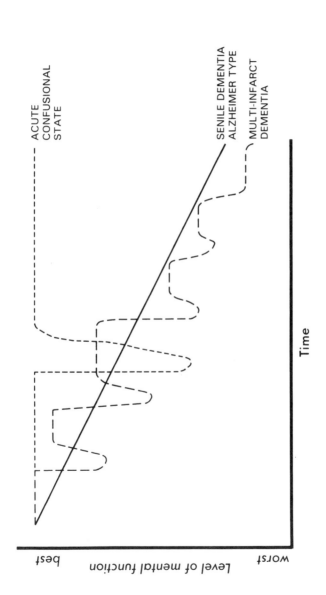

irreversible dementia but, equally important, that when dementia is present the defeatist view that 'nothing can be done' is based on ignorance. By provision of appropriate services and application of appropriate skills, the quality of life of the majority of demented old people can be vastly improved.

Causes of Confusion

Acute Confusional States

Old people, especially if they are already suffering from a mild degree of dementia, are particularly prone to develop acute confusional states. The hallmark of an acute confusional state is sudden onset. The patient's behaviour is often erratic and bizarre and level of awareness of the environment is diminished and fluctuates, often being worse at night. The effect is of perplexity or fear and thoughts and talk are incoherent. Perceptual misinterpretations and hallucinations, especially visual, are common and may result in violent behaviour. Attention and concentration are inhibited and cognitive function is impaired. Focal neuropsychological changes may be a result of the acute confusional state or may point to the underlying pathology. Provided the cause, which is usually physical illness, is detected and is responsive to treatment, then prognosis for recovery of the mental state is good. The time course of acute confusional states is summarised in Figure 5.1. Because of the often serious nature of the underlying illness, nearly half the people admitted to hospital with acute confusional states die before six months have elapsed.[2] Heart failure and infections, especially of the chest and the urinary tract, are probably the commonest causes of acute confusional states in old age. Drugs prescribed by the doctor are also sometimes responsible. Long-acting benzodiazepines and drugs with marked anti-cholinergic effects such as anti-Parkinsonian drugs and some antidepressants are amongst the greatest offenders. Other conditions which can contribute to acute confusional states are summarised in Table 5.1. A special mention should be made of thiamine deficiency. Classically associated with alcoholism and causing an acute confusional state called Wernicke's encephalopathy, characterised by confusion, ophthalmoplegia and ataxia, this deficiency can result in the permanent loss of short-term memory and confabulation (Korsakoff's psychosis). Thiamine deficiency has also been implicated as a cause of prolonged post-operative confusion in elderly patients presented with fractured neck of femur.[5] It is worth considering thiamine supplementation in all acutely ill old people, especially those who may have been taking a poor diet. In patients who are already suffering from dementia, a relatively trivial infection, constipation or change of environment may be sufficient to precipitate an acute worsening of confusion.

Table 5.1: Some Causes of Acute Confusional State

Severe infection	**Systems failures**
chest	cardiac
urine	renal
	hepatic
Metabolic	respiratory embarrassment
diabetes	
thyroid	**Dehydration**
B_{12}	
thiamine	**Intra-cranial**
	stroke
Drugs and toxic	subdural haematoma
carbon monoxide	other space-occupying lesions
alcohol	
anti-cholinergic drugs	**Depressive illness**
benzodiazepines	
(see also Table 2.5 for a fuller list)	

In those otherwise predisposed by dementia (even mild) add:
(change of environment)
constipation
minor infection
pain

The 'reflex diagnosis' of dementia is the greatest enemy of the acutely confused patient and if the onset of confusion is known to be sudden or if it is unknown, then a thorough medical evaluation including a drug history and physical examination is vital. Because of the patient's erratic behaviour and unreliability in taking medication, initial management is usually best in hospital. In most cases, the degree of physical illness will necessitate admission under the care of a physician in geriatric medicine although less ill patients can sometimes be managed on an acute psychiatric ward for old people provided it is on a site with ready access to investigational facilities and medical help. Treatment of the underlying physical illness should be supplemented by appropriate nursing care and general management which may include sedative drugs such as thioridazine. Management will be dealt with in more detail later in this chapter.

Senile Dementia of the Alzheimer Type (SDAT)

This disease affects half of all hospital patients dying with dementia. Women are slightly more likely to develop this disease than men, even allowing for the greater proportion of women in the elderly population.

Clinical. SDAT is characterised by an insidious onset and gradual decline in the mental state (Figure 5.1). Memory difficulties, especially problems in encoding new memories, are usually the first symptoms to be noticed. Often these are attributed at first to absent-mindedness or old age. The onset is so gradual that even a close relative living with the sufferer finds it difficult to put a date on when the patient was last quite normal. In the early stages, previous personality may strongly influence the presentation. The patient who has had a previous tendency to suspiciousness may upset carers by accusing them of stealing misplaced items. The patient with a tendency to dependency may react to these early changes by becoming extremely dependent on relatives, especially if family patterns of behaviour encourage this. Mood disturbance is not, in itself, a feature of SDAT. The patient usually lacks insight and as the disease progresses behaviour may become more erratic. Disorientation for time, place and person will also become more evident. A combination of restlessness (often at its worst in the evening) and topographical disorientation may cause the patient to wander off and get lost. The patient may get up in the early hours of the morning believing she has to get to work or may insist on going 'home' early (even from her own house!) to prepare a meal for the children. Caring relatives find it particularly distressing when the sufferer fails to recognise them. Fortunately, this does not usually happen until a late stage of the disease, but it can be particularly difficult for spouses, especially if an elderly husband is trying to help his wife with personal care and is pushed away by a wife who sees him as a 'strange man'. Spontaneous thought becomes increasingly limited as dementia develops and repetitive talk can become very wearing for carers. Hallucinations are not common unless there is a complicating acute confusional state or there is severe auditory or visual handicap. Rarely, sufferers will find not only other people's faces but also their own faces difficult to recognise. A reflection perceived in a mirror can then give rise to worries that a stranger is in the house. The wife of one of our patients had to take down all mirrors in the house because of this problem. As the disease develops, apraxias may develop in skills such as dressing or washing or the motivation to perform these tasks may fade, further limiting ability to live independently. Incontinence usually develops very late in the course of the disease although it may occur earlier if complicating factors such as poor mobility, inconvenient location of the toilet or urinary tract infection supervene. Dysphasia (see Table 9.1) can lead to frustrating difficulties in communication for both patient and carers. Eventually the point is reached for those living alone where intermittent support is not enough and where admission to an old people's home or hospital for continuing care becomes necessary. Old people living with their families can often continue to live in the community for longer, especially if appropriate support services are offered. Often patients die from other causes before they reach the terminal stage of SDAT though the dementia often seems to contribute to the death. Patients with SDAT usually lose a considerable amount of weight regardless of nutritional intake and an obese patient with advanced dementia is probably not suffering from SDAT. Neurological symptoms develop in the terminal stages of SDAT. By this time patients are often in hospital and may have developed contractures due to inadequate nursing and physiotherapy. At this stage patients need total nursing care. Despite the severity of the patients' handicaps, those who nurse them still often find that they retain emotional responsiveness to their carers.

Aetiology and Pathology. Macroscopically the brains of patients suffering from SDAT are shrunken with widening of the sulci. Microscopically senile plaques are found in the brain in far greater numbers than in ordinary old people.[6] Neuro-fibrillary tangles, found in the hippocampal region of some normal old people, are increased in numbers and more widely distributed especially in earlier-onset cases of SDAT. There may be an accumulation of lipofuscin and granulovacuolar degeneration. The changes are identical with those in presenile dementia of the Alzheimer type although very old patients with SDAT have more localised changes. Biochemical research has shown a markedly reduced level of the cholinergic marker enzyme, acetyl transferase, again more localised in older subjects.[7] Deficiencies in other neurotransmitters have also been found but they are not so marked as in the cholinergic system. There is a genetic component to Alzheimer's disease. Some family pedigrees have been established with dominant inheritance but the genetic contribution to the majority of cases is less clear. An autosomal dominant inheritance with greatly reduced penetrance has been suggested. It can be said that relatives of patients with SDAT have a *slightly* increased risk of developing the disease. It may well be that late-onset SDAT is aetiologically and genetically different from the earlier-onset type.

Diagnosis. The history is the major factor in diagnosis. Insidious onset and a gradual but inexorable progression are the rule. Mental state examination with evidence of memory loss and, in all but the earliest cases, evidence also of impairment in other areas of cortical function such as visuospatial dysfunction and nominal aphasia, confirms the diagnosis. If the patient is seen early in the disease then basic screening tests to exclude metabolic causes of dementia (e.g. B_{12}, thyroid) are indicated. Prominent headaches or focal signs should lead to computerised axial tomography (CAT scan) to exclude space-occupying lesions. CAT scans show the typical brain-shrinkage of SDAT but the overlap with the normal or functionally ill population is too great for this to be of diagnostic use.

Multi-infarct Dementia (MID)

This affects a fifth of psychiatric hospital patients dying with dementia and another fifth have a mixture of SDAT and MID. Men are more commonly affected than women and the 'young old' more than the very elderly.

Clinical. As its name implies, this kind of dementia is asssociated with multiple cerebral infarcts. Onset is therefore usually sudden and the general progression stepwise (Figure 5.1). Often, there is a history of hypertension and there may be frank strokes or other signs of a vascular disease. The patient characteristically retains more insight and often has depression or lability of mood, sometimes with uncontrollable outbursts of emotion ('emotional incontinence'). Performance on psychological testing is more patchy and more variable than for SDAT with a particular tendency to increased confusion at night. Some of these characteristic features have been summed up by Hachinski in his scoring system[8] (Table 5.2) which gives a reasonably reliable differentiation between SDAT and MID and has been confirmed by regional cerebral blood flow and pathological studies.[9] Not all psychological changes associated with stroke are harbingers of dementia and a patient with fluent dysphasia or marked emotional incontinence who is otherwise well preserved may become extremely frustrated if he is labelled or treated as a demented patient.

Aetiology and Pathology. This disease is closely related to stroke illness and is associated with hypertension and atheroma. Most of the lesions are due to atheromatous emboli from extracranial sources. Hopefully measures to reduce the prevalence of hypertension in the population will also reduce the incidence of MID.

On examination the brains of sufferers contain multiple small or

Table 5.2: Ischaemic Score — The Hachinski Scale

Feature	Score
Abrupt onset	2
Stepwise deterioration	1
Fluctuating course	2
Nocturnal confusion	1
Relative preservation of personality	1
Depression	1
Somatic complaints	1
Emotional incontinence	1
History of hypertension	1
History of strokes	2
Evidence of associated atherosclerosis	1
Focal neurological symptoms	2
Focal neurological signs	2

Patients scoring 7 and above may be classified as having multi-infarct dementia, and patients scoring 4 and below may be classified as having primary degenerative dementia.

sometimes large areas of cerebral softening due to infarction. There appears to be a 'threshold effect' with more than 50 ml of softening being associated with clinical dementia.[6]

Diagnosis. Again, this is largely by history and mental state examination. Physical examination may reveal hypertension, focal neurological changes or other signs of vascular insufficiency. A CAT scan is not usually necessary for diagnostic purposes but, where diagnosis is in doubt, it will usually reveal areas of attenuation marking old infarctions.

Other Causes of 'Dementia'

Although other causes of dementia are individually rare, they are important because some cases represent a subacute and potentially reversible confusional state rather than an irreversible dementia. The following list is not complete and the reader is referred to more comprehensive texts[10,11] for a fuller account.

Drugs. The tendency to issue a repeat prescription rather than examine the patient is a great enemy of old people. Many drugs, especially the benzodiazepines and drugs with anti-cholinergic effects, can cause confusion which may be severe enough to precipitate a move from independent living to institutional care.

B₁₂ Deficiency. This is usually, but not always, associated with a megaloblastic anaemia. The patient's mental state may be indistinguishable from SDAT, but an admixture of apparently depressive symptoms, with marked slowing and apathy, can sometimes give a clue. While some patients fail to respond to B_{12} therapy, others show a slow but marked improvement continuing over several months (see Case 5.1).

Folic Acid Deficiency. This is often an incidental finding in demented patients and is only rarely of aetiological significance. Treatment with folic acid, which is cheap and may produce some benefit, is probably justified until diet can be improved.

Thyroid Deficiency. Coarsening of the hair, a 'puffy' facial appearance, pre-tibial myxoedema and a deep voice may be noted but are not always present. The changes of hypothyroidism are sometimes so insidious that they are mistaken for 'normal ageing' and when mental changes supervene, they are attributed to SDAT. Marked slowing and apathy are again characteristic, but treatment with thyroxine often partially or fully restores mental function.

Subudural Haematoma. Chronic subdural haematoma is notoriously difficult to diagnose before death. A high index of suspicion is essential and if there is a history of head injury or if the level of consciousness is varying markedly, an expert opinion and CAT scan is justified.

Other Space-occupying Lesion. Unexplained mental symptoms are sometimes due to intra-cranial growths. If these are malignant, they are often aggressive and declare themselves quickly. They are also often inoperable. Slow-growing, benign meningiomas can often mimic mental illness and a parasaggital meningioma can produce a picture quite similar to that of normal-pressure hydrocephalus.

Normal-pressure Hydrocephalus. This is characterised by the triad of confusion, abnormal gait and incontinence, more severe than would be expected in an early dementia. Patients presenting with this triad should be referred early for specialist assessment as the insertion of a shunt can sometimes reverse the disability.

Alcoholic Dementia. The single greatest risk factor amongst heavy drinkers for developing alcoholic dementia is increasing age. Disinhibition and impaired judgement are more common early in this form of dementia than in SDAT. Its progress may be arreseted by abstention from alcohol. It may also be an accelerating factor in the deterioration due to MID or SDAT. A history of excessive alcohol intake may be hard to elicit but hard-drinking friends or relatives, unexplained macrocytic anaemia or abnormal liver function tests may provide a clue.

Neurosyphilis. This is now a very rare cause of dementia in old age, but should not be discounted, especially if there is a relevant past history or if the clinical picture is atypical.

Depressive Pseudo-dementia. This is not really a true *diagnostic term* but serves as a useful reminder that some severely depressed patients, especially those with profound psychomotor retardation, may appear to be intellecutally impaired and may perform badly on memory tests. A history of relatively rapid onset, with loss of interest rather than loss of memory as the first symptom, and a positive personal or family history of affective illness are useful pointers.

'Cortical' and 'Subcortical' Dementia

There is a new emphasis on the clinical distinction between cortical and subcortical dementia. Alzheimer's dementia is the classic cortical dementia with marked aphasia, amnesia and impaired judgement. The subcortical dementias include the toxic and metabolic dementias and are characterised by forgetfulness, marked psychomotor slowing, apathetic or depressed mood, and often by abnormal posture, muscle tone and movements. Multi-infarct dementia often produces a 'mixed' picture. The terms 'cortical' and 'subcortical' are probably anatomically misleading owing to the complicated interactions of systems within the brain. Nevertheless, they are clinically relevant, especially as so-called subcortical features can be an important clue to a potentially treatable dementia.

Case 5.1:

Mrs J.W. was an 83-year-old married woman who lived with her husband. About six years before presentation she had been admitted to a psychiatric ward with apparent depression. She was seen at home by a psychiatrist where she was in bed, almost stuperose, and apparently confused. Her husband said that she had been more or less normal until six weeks ago when she had started to deteriorate. A presumptive diagnosis of depressive pseudo-dementia was made but on admission she was found to have a profound megaloblastic anaemia

Figure 5.2: Flow Chart for Diagnosis of Some Important Causes of Confusion

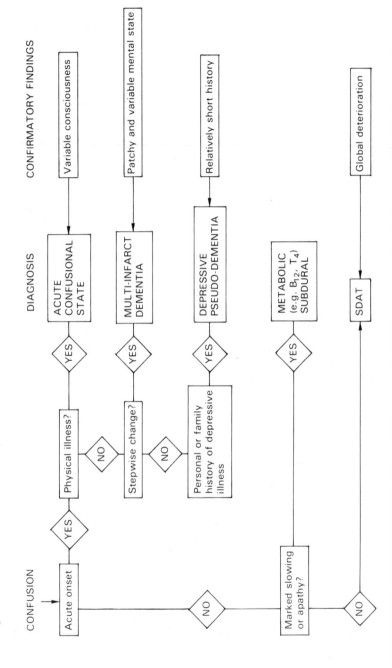

with a B_{12} deficiency. Her mental state gradually improved with B_{12} injections but her memory is still far from perfect. However, when she was last seen at home, when the district nurse was mentioned to her, she was able to find the drawer where the vials of neo-cytamen (B_{12}) were kept.

Not all confusion is due to irreversible dementia, and not all mental slowing is due to depression. Figure 5.2 is a flow chart for the diagnosis of some of the most important causes of confusion.

Management

Specific psychological and pharmacological approaches will be discussed in Chapters 8, 9 and 10. This section discusses the general approach to the problem of confusion. It is vital that the professional helper tries to understand how the patient experiences the problem. Patients, however confused, will have some residual abilities. In their attempt to make sense of the situation they find themselves in, they may cling to some inappropriate idea, for example, that they have to go home to make tea for the children. In an acute confusional state the patient may also feel frightened and threatened by attempts to help. The confused patient may easily be made anxious by changes in environment and, in an attempt at self-preservation, may adopt a very restricted life-style that resists intervention by would-be helpers.

Analysing the Problem

Figure 5.3 presents an interactive model of confusion. This stresses that factors in the brain, the internal environment, the special senses and the external environment may all interact to cause confusion. In any one patient the contribution of environmental and personal factors will be unique and even where there is irreversible brain damage, attention to such factors as constipation, a malfunctioning hearing aid and enviromental design, may produce marked improvement. Brain intrinsic factors and factors in the internal environment have already been discussed; special senses , the external environment and some specific points in management will be considered in the remainder of this chapter.

Special Senses

Sensory deprivation is used in 'brain-washing' and interrogation techniques to produce confusion and disorientation. Those of us who are

Figure 5.3: An Interactive Model of 'Confusion'

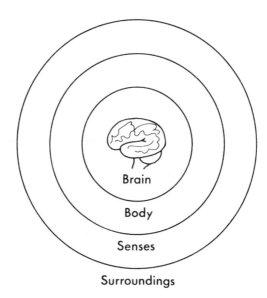

blessed with good sight and hearing forget how confusing and frightening the world can be for an old person with poor hearing or eyesight. Disabilities in the special senses can combine with defects in other systems to render the old person extremely vulnerable. Imagine trying to cross a busy road with misty glasses, ear plugs and your ankles hobbled and you will get some idea of the predicament some old people find themselves in.

External Environment

Change of environment can provoke or worsen confusion, especially if badly managed. If an old person who is confused has to be subjected to a change of environment, for example an acute hospital admission or entering residential care, it is vital that the change is carefully managed. The old person should be prepared in advance. A familiar person should accompany her. As the transition proceeds, the person should be reminded what is happening and where she is. Unfortunately, many old people enter residential care or hospital in crisis without adequate management of the change and an unnecessary increase in confusion occurs. The external environment can also be used 'prosthetically'. A shopping list is a simple example of a memory prosthesis but the same principle lies behind labels such as 'remember to lock the door before you go to bed', 'only cook a meal for one person' and telephone calls 'Hello Mum; it's time to get up. The day-centre ambulance will be calling soon' which can be extremely helpful to the mildly demented. In institutions, careful design and labelling can make toilets more easily recognisable and accessible and reduce incontinence. Questions of environmental design will be discussed more fully in Chapter 9.

Reality Orientation

This was the first psychological approach suggested specifically for use with the 'confused' elderly, and it has been influential in changing the prevailing ethos that nothing could be done for this group of people. Developed in the late 1950s, it emphasised two important aspects of the management of confused elderly people that had hitherto been neglected. First, that the confused elderly person has the same rights of dignity, respect and independence within their remaining capabilities as anyone else. The aim here was to make professionals aware of the dehumanising aspects of institutional practices. Not only do such practices lead to a rapid deterioration of the confused person's preserved abilities, but they have the quality of being self-fulfilling prophecies: they create the behavioural problems which can then be used to justify the inhumane conditions. Secondly, it was suggested as a way of reducing the confused person's disorientation, and therefore encouraging more appropriate behaviour. To achieve this, staff are trained to orientate the confused person regularly to time, place and person in a relaxed and unthreatening manner. This can be carried out either in regular small groups, or routinely during every interaction (24-hour reality orientation).

Although more recently reality orientation has been subject to a number of criticisms, these have often been based on misconceptions, such as the belief that because it is not a cure, it is no use. In fact, much successful practice in medicine is based not on cure, but rather on providing some permanent prosthesis to reduce the effects of a particular difficulty. With reality orientation in its broader form, Holden and Woods[12] provide a sound and practical approach from which to meet the psychological needs of a confused elderly person.

Reminiscence

It has been suggested that as old age is reached, all elderly people review their lives, and that encouraging this facilitates the evaluation, understanding and acceptance of their lives. A number of reminiscence tape-slide packs have been produced, which through the use of the sights and sounds taken from everyday life in a specific period (e.g. the war years) stimulate the sharing of reminiscences between elderly people in small group settings. The therapist gradually moves focus away from himself, towards allowing the elderly individuals to take control of the session, and interact amongst themselves. There is no doubt that such an approach allows the elderly person to see the value of her own life and care staff to see the elderly person in a new light, as a valued individual. It also increases the probability of the participants getting to know each other. This final aspect of reminiscence suggests the potentially important use in community settings, such as sheltered flats. Because the physical effects of ageing inhibit the development of new relationships, moving into such accommodation can leave the elderly individual as isolated as she was before. Reminiscence used as the focus for bringing together residents in such community facilities can foster the development of relationships between elderly individuals who might go on living next to each other, isolated, for a number of years.

A final note of caution must be sounded regarding reminiscence. Although included in this chapter on confusion, reminiscence by itself should only be used with elderly people with little or no confusion. One study has shown that a group of confused elderly people receiving regular reminiscence for one month prior to reality orientation did markedly less well than a group receiving reality orientation first of all.[13] Also, when there is marked confusion, reminiscing by itself may increase the level of confusion.

The Personal Touch

Every elderly confused person faces a unique set of problems and has a unique set of experiences to help her cope. The logical analysis of problems helps. Even if the diagnosis is dementia, treating constipation, putting a battery in the hearing aid or developing a regular routine including appropriate social support can work wonders. The relatives also deserve special consideration. In addition to the strains imposed by problems of incontinence, wandering or unpredictable behaviour, they may face the emotional stress of 'living bereavement' and be worn down by the needs for 24-hour care, 365 days a year. They need practical help such as arranging attendance allowance or day care but often they also need emotional support such as can be provided by a relatives' support group run by professionals or by a voluntary body such as the Alzheimer's Disease Society.

Drugs

There is no drug yet discovered which can arrest the progress of SDAT

Figure 5.4: Management of Insomnia in an Elderly Confused
Patient

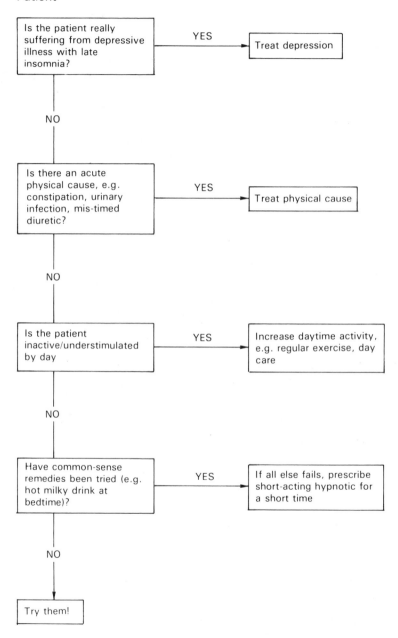

or MID or reliably produce clinically significant improvement in the mental state of patients suffering from these diseases. The discovery that the cholinergic neurotransmitter systems are particularly affected in Alzheimer's disease led to a search for a 'replacement therapy' analagous to the use of L-dopa in Parkinson's disease. Choline and its precursor lecithin have been given to demented patients but the results have been generally disappointing. Anti-cholinesterase drugs and cholinergic agonists have also been tried without any major success as yet. Other drugs have been marketed as cerebral metabolic enhancers but, although in the experimental situation they have shown marginal benefit, in the clinical situation this is rarely significant. The search continues for drugs to help this group of patients but at present there is no specific treatment.

Symptomatic treatment with drugs should be avoided if possible because of the risk of adverse effects. If an elderly confused patient is restless at night, this can be the last straw for caring relatives. Nevertheless, other approaches should be tried before drugs. This is illustrated in Figure 5.4. Wandering is a common problem. Really it is a group of problems. Some demented patients wander in a fairly reliable and safe way around their home or institution and should be allowed to do so. Others are a danger to themselves and other people and the wandering has to be controlled. If common-sense measures (e.g. more directed exercise, other occupation or treating constipation) fail then drugs have to be used. Thioridazine is a neuroleptic often used in old people because of its relative lack of side effects and its use and other drugs which may be used to control disturbed behaviour are discussed in Chapter 10.

Other Measures.

The practice of medicine is more than the prescription of drugs. Relatives of demented patients often complain that the disease has not been explained to them and that they did not know what to expect. Sometimes relatives, especially spouses, will go through a period of 'living bereavement'. The demented relative is so changed that it is as if he or she were dead. Appropriate counselling can be a great help at this stage and is a role that various professionals may be trained to take. At other times, illness in old age will expose stresses that have been present in a marriage for many years. Again, this may be amenable to a counselling approach.

Practical help is also needed. Doctors should let appropriate relatives know about the availability of financial help in the form of attendance allowance and also about social services and how to contact the local social services office. Social workers can often offer practical and emotional support to elderly ill people and their relatives. With so many different professionals potentially involved, good communication is vital. When it can be done without breach of confidence, copying of relevant letters to different professionals involved can be an economical way of achieving this. Involving social workers in informal case conferences, ideally face to face, but sometimes over the telephone, can break down prejudice between professions and improve co-operative management. The telephone is often a great ally both for gathering and disseminating relevant information. Sadly, statutory community services are very variable. Whereas in some places the home help service or the district nurse may be able to attend two mornings or more a week to ensure the patient is ready for the day centre or the day hospital, in other areas none of these services will be available. The availability and quality of hospital-based services are also variable.

Conclusion

In this chapter we have adopted an interactive model for the understanding of confused old people. We have looked at the way in which physical, psychological and environmental factors can interact to generate or worsen confusion. We have stressed that, even when confusion is due to an irreversible dementia, there may well be modifications that can be made in other areas to improve the patient's function and quality of life. We have argued that good health and social care for confused old people is a measure of the quality of our civilisation and, sadly, at present is a measure which finds us wanting.

Notes

1. Wells, N.E.J., *Dementia in Old Age* (Office of Health Economics, London, 1979).

2. Blessed, G. and Wilson, I.D. 'The Contemporary Natural History of Mental Disorder in Old Age', *British Journal of Psychiatry,* 141, 1982, 59–67.

3. BMJ Leader. 'Dementia, the Quiet Epidemic', *British Medical Journal,* 1978, 1, 1–2

4. Dick, D.H., *The Rising Tide: Developing Services for Mental Illness in Old Age,* (NHS Health Advisory Service, Sutton, 1982).

5. Older, M.W.J. and Dickerson, J.W.T., 'Thiamine and the Elderly Orthopaedic Patient', *Age and Ageing,* 11, 1982, 101–7.

6. Blessed, G., Tomlinson, B.E. and Roth, M., 'The Association between Quantitative Measures of Dementia and Senile Change in the Grey Matter of Elderly People', *British Journal of Psychiatry,* 144, 1968, 797–811.

7. Rossor, M.N., Iversen, L.L., Reynolds, G.P., Mountjoy, C.Q., and Roth, M., 'Neurochemical Characteristics of Early and Late Onset Types of Alzheimer's Disease', *British Medical Journal,* 288, 1984, 961–4.

8. Hachinski, V.C., Illiff, L.D., Zilka, E. Du Bonlay, G.H., McAllister, V.L., Marshall, J., Russell, R.W.R. and Symon, L., 'Cerebral Blood Flow in Dementia', *Archives of Neurology*, 32, 1975, 632–7.

9. Rosen, W.G., Terry, R.D., Fuld, P.A., Katzman, R. and Peck, A. 'Pathological Verification of Ischemic Score in Differentiation of Dementias', *Annals of Neurology*, 7, 1980, 5, 486–8.

10. Lishman, W.A., *Organic Psychiatry*, (Blackwell Scientific Publications, London, 1978).

11. Cummings, J.L. and Benson, D.F., *Dementia, A Clinical Approach*, (Butterworth, Boston, 1983).

12. Holden, U.P. and Woods, R.T., *Reality Orientation: Psychological Approaches to the Confused Elderly*, (Churchill Livingstone, London, 1982).

13. Baines, S., Saxby, P. and Ehlert, K., 'Reality Orientation and Reminiscence Therapy: A Controlled Cross Over Study of Elderly Confused People', unpublished, 1984, available from Mr P. Saxby, Department of Clinical Psychology, Moorhaven Hospital, Ivybridge, Devon, PL21 0EX.

6 HYPOCHONDRIASIS

Nearly everyone who is reading this sentence will, after a moment's thought, be able to isolate some area of mild discomfort or pain in their own body. Indeed it is estimated that some three out of four people have symptoms in any given month which lead them to take a clear response such as medicating themselves, resting in bed or visiting their GPs. However, most of us do not let the presence of mild pain or discomfort interfere with our leisure activities or work: we limit our outward expression of this and easily accept reassurance from friends, relatives or a doctor. A few individuals do not respond easily to such reassurance. They are convinced that they are physically ill, present an amount of distress and pain disproportionate to any organic disease which might be present and assiduously pursue medical care with repeatedly unsuccessful results: the term hypochondriasis is used to describe this presentation. Some will present a hypochondriacal complaint for which no physical cause can be found, others have not only a hypochondriacal complaint but also an unfounded belief that they are suffering from a specific illness, a hypochondriacal conviction (delusion). Elderly people who are hypochondriacal sometimes show a degree and type of distressed behaviour which is not only difficult for friends and relatives, but also presents apparently insurmountable problems to the doctor and other professionals. There seem to be a number of related factors arising during the process of ageing which might account for this.

As individuals get older there will be an increasing build-up of minor physical lesions which can become the focus of the hypochondriacal complaint. Not only this, they will have more direct experience of those close to them suffering serious or terminal illnesses. Such experiences can heighten anxiety directly, by raising fears of death, and indirectly, by increasing isolation from meaningful relationships. Where the level of anxiety is raised there is a real danger that minor aches and pains can be perceived as serious illness. It is not unusual to find the site of the hypochondriacal complaint as having a minor physical lesion, or being of the same kind as the terminal illness which a close relative suffered.

A recent review of emotion in relation to the elderly suggests that once an emotion has been aroused it may persist for a longer period of time.[1] If this is the case then as we will see later it is easy to understand the persistence of hypochondriacal fear once it has arisen in the elderly person.

89

As will be seen in Chapters 8 and 9, because of various changes, for example reduction of physical capacity and loss of earning ability, elderly people become more dependent on their environment. The importance of this dependence on family members or caring neighbours should not be underestimated. Younger people are much more able to remove themselves from unsatisfactory or distressing relationships. Elderly people who are experiencing such distressing relationships may be unwilling or unable to remove themselves from the situation, and indeed may be dependent in some important way on the person they find difficult.

Similarly an elderly person who suffers from a poor social network, or a very low level of perceived emotional contact with important family members, can find that the sick role brings with it a sudden and dramatic increase in time and interest from others. Becoming 'well' again can mean the 'loss' of relationships the elderly person has come to depend on. In a few instances visits from family members can be contingent only upon 'real' physical illness as the family do not believe in anxiety or depression.

Assessment of the Hypochondriacal Presentation

Clinical studies suggest that hypochondriasis should not be viewed as a unitary syndrome, but as a phenomenon which is frequently associated with a treatable psychiatric or medical state.[2] The first step in the effective management of elderly people with hypochondriacal complaints is the identification and treatment of such illnesses.

Physical Illness

Reaching a diagnosis which rests on the absence of positive signs of physical illness rather than confirmatory signs is always a risky business. A retrospective view of the diagnostic category of hysteria and the dramatic levels of misdiagnosis of people with serious organic illness, highlights this difficulty for the clinician. Physical illness and psychiatric disorder can appear together, especially in the elderly person where multiple pathology is frequent.[3] Once a patient is labelled as hypochondriacal there is a danger that because she has had one complete examination recently the doctor assumes that subsequent complaints are hypochondriacal in nature: the patient cries wolf once too often! In one case a 67-year-old woman living alone with her brother was diagnosed as having pneumonia by one of the authors during a psychiatric domiciliary visit requested by the GP. Her hypochondriasis pre-dated the pneumonia and continued after the pneumonia responded to treatment. After a number of months of difficult management characterised by non-compliance to antidepressant therapy she accepted and fully responded to a full course of ECT. In summary, then, the elderly person is more at risk from the appearance of a new serious illness and this may appear at any time before, during or after any management programme implemented by the psychiatric team.

Affective Disorder

After a full physical investigation and with continued monitoring of physical state, the next step is to ascertain whether or not the hypochondriasis is part of an affective disorder. There is a clear and strong association between hypochondriasis and affective disorder. De Alaracon found that nearly two-thirds of 152 consecutive depressed patients admitted to a geriatric unit had hypochondriacal symptoms.[4] The importance of identifying the elderly person who presents with hypochondriasis as part of a depressive illness cannot be over-stressed, not just because there are effective treatments for depression, but because of the high risk of suicide attempts (over a third in De Alaracon's study) in depressed elderly people who show hypochondriasis as the dominant symptom.

Digestive symptoms, ranging from intense over-concern about constipation to delusions about the cessation of bowel movement and about head and facial pain, are by far the most frequent hypochondriacal symptoms associated with depression in the aged.[4,5] Other preoccupations may concern cardiovascular, urinary and genital areas of the body. Complaints about skin and hair, for example that handfulls of hair are falling out, seem to largely be confined to women. From the authors' own experience the identification of a depressive illness masquerading as a hypochondriasis is difficult in some cases. The doctor needs to assess, through direct questioning, the patient's mood and mental state, looking for the presence of sleep disturbance, depressive thoughts, suicidal ideas and loss of energy and interest in life, family, work and hobbies. The recent, rapid onset of hypochondriacal symptoms in a person who has never previously had such symptoms, should be regarded as a possible indicator of affective disorder. Where an elderly person has shown lifelong hypochondriacal behaviour with a fondness for unnecessary medication, etc., a depressive episode may be signalled by a dramatic change in intensity of her concern or in the nature and content of her worries. Of all patients, those who have hypochondriacal complaints concerning facial or head pain are the most likely to show an atypical presentation of a depressive illness.[6]

Where uncertainty exists as to the presence or not of a depressive illness, any intervention, whether psychological or physical, should be based on a testable hypothesis about the nature and causes of the hypochondriasis, should be time limited, and should be used as an assessment of the nature of the disorder. For example, in a married couple, it is not always easy to assess the degree to which the hypochondriacal complaints arise from marital arguments through the exacerbation of anxiety, rather than arising out of a depressive illness which then undermines a fragile marital harmony. As has been emphasised in other chapters the possibility of successful treatment can be maximised through the use of carefully planned and timed interventions considering all the relevant physical, psychiatric, psychological and social factors. Figure 6.1 summarises the steps which should be taken in the treatment of a patient with hypochondriacal complaints.

Management of the Hypochondriacal Patient

The Depressed Hypochondriac

Many of those depressed patients with predominant hypochondriasis show particularly poor compliance with physical psychiatric treatments, perhaps because they believe they are not being treated appropriately. Thus a clear and co-ordinated management plan, a necessary condition for any good psychiatric practice, becomes of paramount importance in these cases. At its core should be a consistent response by the psychiatric team to make the acceptance of a necessary physical treatment for depression more, rather than less, likely. A pattern of repeated admission and discharge during which the person never complies adequately with any treatment offered should be resisted. Admission should normally only take place with the agreement of the patient to a clear contract to accept a particular treatment, not because, for example, the spouse cannot cope any longer with the partner's complaints. Whilst coercion is generally undesirable, the alternative may be to leave the elderly person in distress for months at a time because the hypochondriacal behaviour prevents the implementation of effective physical treatment. Since the GP may receive the butt of the hypochondriacal complaints, he must be kept fully informed of the psychiatric team's management plan.

The case-history presented next illustrates how the initial psychological intervention failed to make a significant change in a woman who had a depressive hypochondriasis. However, this paved the way for decisions about her management which led to her eventually accepting the

Figure 6.1: Simplified Flow Chart Showing the Steps Involved in Treating the Hypochondriacal Patient

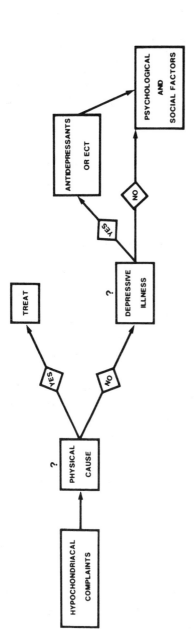

appropriate physical treatment.

Case 6.1:

Mrs F.V. was a 67-year-old married woman who was taken over by our team one month after being discharged from a psychiatric ward where incomplete treatment with antidepressants, one application of ECT and attempts at marital therapy had failed. She had a three-year history of physical complaints apparently precipitated by having her ears pierced and previous physical investigations included a nose biopsy. Interestingly her main presenting symptom was of pain in her nose but included ear and mouth pain, chest pain, swollen ankles, athlete's foot and worries about her diabetes for which she received a daily injection from a district nurse. Figure 6.2 gives an outline of treatment attempted with Mrs F.V. and illustrates well the difficulties caused for all concerned by poor compliance. It was 'catch 22' for the staff involved: on the one hand Mrs F.V. demanded help for her physical condition, yet every treatment attempt made whether it was antidepressant medication, pain killers or soothing ear drops resulted in an apparent exacerbation of her symptoms, presumably because of her hypersensitivity to small changes in her bodily state and then non-compliance.

Mrs F.V.'s ambivalence towards medication led to initial attempts at a psychological intervention. Marital work was impossible because of Mrs F.V.'s preoccupation with her physical state which was occasionally interspersed with heated arguments with her husband and individual work with Mr F.V. to try to reduce the level of his expressed anger and increase his coping skills failed because of his inability to comply. As he put it, he could cope much better at Dunkirk with his friends being killed around him than with his wife in this condition.

Two admissions ensued both of which were characterised by lack of compliance and after her discharge from the second admission the team agreed to resist further admissions until she consented to a full course of ECT. There was a gradual and eventually very marked change in Mrs F.V. over eleven ECT's. Her complaints diminished, although she still reported some ear and mouth pain, and her level of interest and activity greatly increased. After the sixth ECT marital work was again instituted with the aim of preparing Mr and Mrs F.V. for a resumption in normal life, as Mr F.V. had taken over most of his wife's role as a housewife. Also, ways in which both could express their affection more directly to each other were explored, and

Figure 6.2: Overview of Mrs F.V.'s Treatment

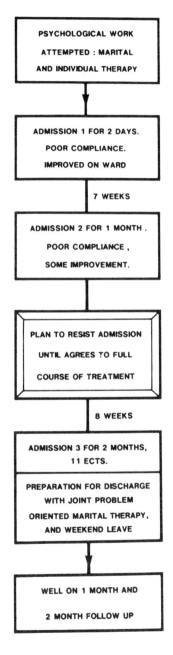

nursing staff encouraged Mrs F.V. to be more independent regarding her physical health by teaching her to self-administer her insulin. Mr and Mrs F.V. did not wish to attend regularly for marital work after her discharge, but Mrs F.V. maintained her improvement at two-month follow-up. A year later she relapsed, following a physical illness, but readily agreed to come into hospital for a course of ECT and maintenance antidepressants, to which she responded rapidly and completely.

Psychological Factors

As with all psychiatric phenomena psychological factors will be relevant whether or not any physical therapies are being carried out. Whilst there are a common set of psychological factors which may be influencing the elderly person's hypochondriacal complaints, the relative importance of these factors may differ between individuals and the management plans may also be quite different. Indeed, management plans based on different theoretical models might have to be used with different individuals. Although it is beyond the scope of this book to explore this in detail, two broadly different kinds of approach will be discussed next.

Chronic Illness Behaviour

The elderly person who has shown a life-long pattern of illness behaviour, who is often taking a number of inappropriate and possibly harmful medicines, presents particular difficulties for psychiatric services. These patients have often either failed to respond to traditional physical psychiatric treatments, or refused to have anything to do with psychiatry because they believe their problems are physical!

It can be almost impossible to discover what psychological factors were present 30 or 40 years ago to cause the problem to develop. Indeed even if they can be identified they may have little bearing on the current situation. There is growing evidence that the responses, of the carers involved, to the illness behaviour may be crucial in the maintenance or improvement of these difficulties. For example, one study of married chronic pain patients showed that a reduction of attention by the spouses to their pain behaviour resulted in significantly lower levels of reported pain.[7]

The importance of carers' actions and verbal responses to any person with chronic psychological difficulties is discussed in more detail in Chapter 9 and interested readers are referred to a more detailed account of the behavioural treatment of chronic illness behaviour by Wooley, Blackwell and Winget (1978).[8] A case illustrating the psychological management of an elderly person presenting with such behaviour is presented next.

Case 6.2:

Mrs C.F. was a 77-year-old divorced woman living on her own who was visited three or four times a week by her caring stepdaughter. Mrs C.F.'s husband, who had left her a number of years previously because of her illness behaviour, lived nearby and had developed dementia. She had a long history of taking to her bed as a means of coping and indeed, during her marriage, a housekeeper had been employed because of her failure to take on this role. She was diagnosed as having a neurotic depression and the community nurse asked the clinical psychologist to become involved because of difficulty in being able to help. Because of the resentment shown by Mrs C.F. to the community nurse and psychiatrist, and the high level of care and involvement shown by the stepdaughter, it was decided that it might be more constructive and effective to decide on a treatment plan which the stepdaughter could carry out. She had already developed a planned week which involved sharing her time between her stepmother, father, own family and part-time job! She was particularly concerned at what she regarded as the wasted life her stepmother was leading and how her preoccupation with her physical state had driven away most remaining social contacts. The stepdaughter was extremely pleased to have a specific plan to work from as she felt she never knew how best to cope with her stepmother's behaviour. The main points of the plan are presented in Table 6.1 and it involved her redistributing her time and care to reinforce more appropriate aspects of her stepmother's behaviour. A further aim was to reduce the antagonism which the stepmother's behaviour generated in the stepdaughter. Thus the stepdaughter was given verbal strategies which allowed her to state clearly her care for her stepmother, even in the most aggravating situations such as a middle-of-the-night call-out, without reinforcing these aspects of her stepmother's behaviour. Over a six-week period on a 10-point rating scale (with 10 representing the worst illness behaviour and 0 representing no illness behaviour) the stepdaughter's average rating per week changed from 7.5 to 5.0, indicating a definite improvement. This was further confirmed by a visit two months later by the psychiatrist who found her mental state 'much improved'. This improvement has continued nine months later even though the step

Table 6.1: Mrs C.F.'s Problems and Treatment Approach

Problem	Solution
Resents visit by psychiatrist/psychologist	Intervene through caring stepdaughter
Constant talk about physical state	Reduct time and input associated with this
Little normal conversation	Time and interest increased when this produced
Infrequent self and house-care activity	Increase encouragement or reinforcement for attempts at particular activities
Lack of insight about constant talk of physical symptoms	When complaints above a certain level stepdaughter leaves, after explaining reason why
Suicidal/severe illness behaviour, e.g. heart attack phone calls at 2.00 a.m.	Stepdaughter visits stepmother but limits stay to 1 min. if no evidence of illness

daughter has had to reduce the time spent with her stepmother because of her father's increasing confusion and disability. It is interesting that behavioural change took place more slowly than the change in Mrs C.F.'s verbal behaviour. Thus the stepdaughter noticed her stepmother talking less about her physical state and being aware of and stopping herself in mid-stream of physical complaints saying to the stepdaughter, for example, 'But you don't want to hear about that do you', prior to her taking up various household tasks again. Facilitating self-help behaviour is a common problem where there is little self-help behaviour to start with and it is tempting for relatives, with only a limited amount of time, to do the household tasks anyway. Also relatives can find poor performance hard to tolerate and might not regard this necessary step forward as a step at all!

It is unfortunate that such an approach is not adopted in a more general way by services. These are usually geared towards reinforcing illness behaviour; The GP health visitor or community nurse only visiting and spending more time with the hypochondriacal elderly person when she presents as ill, rather than after a period in which she does not present as ill.

Anxiety and Anxiety Reduction

Hypochondriacal complaints are as commonly associated with anxiety as they are with depression. This is not surprising as raised anxiety usually heightens the experience of pain, and the experience of pain can induce anxiety resulting in a self-maintaining loop: a vicious circle. Figure 6.3 is a simplified model of hypochondriasis based on this idea. It can be seen, then, that reducing the elderly person's level of anxiety directly or indirectly will break this vicious circle and reduce the experience of physical symptoms, which should in turn lead to an abatement of the hypochondriacal complaints.

Figure 6.3: Simplified Model of Hypochondriasis Illustrating the Role of Anxiety

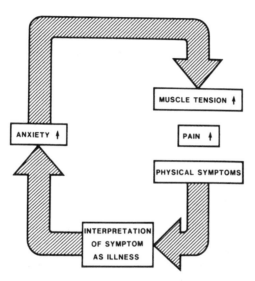

There may be a quite different set of factors contributing to each elderly individual's anxiety (see Figure 6.4). These contributory factors must be identified and their relative importance evaluated. Information will need to be gathered from careful interviews with the patient and involved family members or supporters. Where someone is reluctant or apparently unable to give much detail about everyday circumstances a great deal of information can often be gathered by the detailed review of an average day, from waking up in the morning to going to bed at night. How the complaints affect this average day can give information about what might be raising anxiety, how the patients cope with their symptoms and what kind of social contacts and interests they have. Psychological interviews such as this differ from diagnostic interviews because they do not try to fit the client's experiences into a psychiatric diagnosis, but rather the aim is to understand the client's perception of

Figure 6.4: Factors Exacerbating Anxiety in the Elderly Person Showing Hypochondriasis

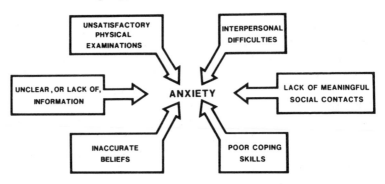

what is happening to her and help her make sense of, and eventually control, her unpleasant experiences.

Information, Explanation and Examination. Elderly people presenting in a state of anxiety in any medical setting may easily misinterpret or forget what is being said to them. Information should be kept simple and if possible written down. One important aspect of information simplification is the avoidance of technical terms. This can be illustrated by referring to one study on beliefs about peptic ulcer formation, which found that whilst most patients had a clear idea that acid was important in ulcer formation, only 10 per cent had realised that acid was secreted by the stomach, some thinking it came from the teeth when food was chewed and others from the brain when food was swallowed.[9] It is also likely that elderly patients will have some other minor discomforts which often have impressive labels, for example sinusitis or gastritis. These may be misunderstood as being the reason for their hypochondriacal complaints, and their possible implications should be simply explained and clarified.

Whenever there is a 'genuine' physical illness, in a patient who also has hypochondriacal complaints, the emphasis should again be on clarity of explanation and treatment approach. However, despite the best efforts of the physician, this may be a frustrating experience, as even the mildest of side effects arising from treatment may be magnified out of all proportion, because of the patients' hypersensitivity to changes in their own body state. Invasive tests are particularly risky in this respect, and the physician should be fully aware of the possible consequences of such testing. Whenever possible the elderly person should be encouraged to cope with her particular illness as far as is reasonable to expect. As we saw in Case 6.1 from being dependent on a district nurse for her insulin injection, Mrs F.V. was taught to self-administer her insulin and monitor her urine sugar level.

One common area of misunderstanding by staff is the hypochondriacal patients' experience of pain. Thus patients will be told they are 'imagining' the pain because there is no physical lesion or that the pain is psychological. In fact pain is a subjective experience and as such should be accepted as being real for the patient who reports it.[10] Comments like those just mentioned can only undermine a therapeutic relationship, isolating the person by attempting to invalidate her experience. Educating the psychiatric team in developing a common understanding and approach towards particular problems such as this is an important task in developing true multidisciplinary team work.

There is some evidence that examination on request (within reason) when carried out promptly and thoroughly in response to acute hypochondriacal fears is helpful, although the reassurance given may not persist for very long. The real danger, especially for the overworked GP, is that persistent calls result in the GP giving a rushed examination, not listening to the expressed fears, or even getting angry. More harm than good will be done if this happens. Physical examination should be thorough and *appear* to be thorough to the patient. Saying in a gentle tone of voice 'I can understand that you feel you are ill but there is really not anything seriously wrong with you' is far better than entering into any kind of persuasive argument with the patient which will only raise her anxiety level still further and exacerbate her physical symptoms. It is not perhaps so surprising that people find it hard to accept reassurance from doctors when even today many patients with serious or terminal illness are neither informed nor counselled about their condition, despite the fact that studies indicate most people would rather have such information than not.

In summary, then, clarity and simplicity of information, and prompt physical examinations at reasonable intervals with reassurance, will help to reduce anxiety and may reduce the level of hypochondriacal complaints. Psychotherapeutic approaches which have emphasised such aspects of treatment have shown promising results.[11] Even when the hypochondriasis is part of a depressive illness this approach is important at the very least because it facilitates the patient's trust and confidence which will improve compliance with any necessary treatment.

Beliefs, Expectations and Behaviour. The degree to which we believe certain things affect the level of emotion experienced. Thus if a person has a 95 per cent belief she has a serious illness such as cancer, she will feel a great deal of anxiety. However, such a belief may be erroneous, for example resulting from a misinterpretation of the physiological components of anxiety. This kind of selective perception by elderly people can operate in a wider way so that they may deny or exclude evidence which is contradictory to their strongly held belief that they are seriously ill. Whilst it may be possible with skilled and empathic questioning to encourage the consideration of alternative explanations for their experiences, it is often much more effective to set up a test of the reality of their beliefs.

Case 6.3:

Mrs I.D. was a 69-year-old woman who presented with abdominal pains and a conviction these pains were the result of cancer. A depressive hypochondriasis was diagnosed and her reponse to monoamine oxidase inhibitors was dramatic, but despite this she failed to take these antidepressants on discharge and quickly relapsed. In addition to looking at the problem of compliance within therapeutic sessions, it was clear on discharge that she still had some erroneous beliefs regarding her health. Thus despite the GP weighing her regularly, she was convinced she was losing weight and hence had a serious illness. When she discovered the therapist was interested in finding out what was really happening, she readily agreed to a 'reality test'. Thus she was to *self-monitor* her own weight and bring it in to each session for the therapist to record. As part of this, it was explained that she would need to use the same weighing machine, wear similar clothing, and to expect a 2 lb fluctuation because of fluid balance. Within the space of three or four weeks she agreed that in fact she wasn't losing weight and hence we were able to explore further how erroneous beliefs such as this and, for example, regarding her medication could actually adversely affect her health. Eventually through becoming more socially active, she developed a close relationship with a man and was helped through some of her anxiety about becoming sexually active again for the first time since the death of her second husband. There were no further problems with medication compliance.

As we will see in another chapter, a person's beliefs will influence her behaviour and vice versa. Looking at this inter-relationship and its consequences on a person's emotional state is the basis of cognitive therapy which has been validated as an effective psychological approach to the treatment of depression.

The importance of self-monitoring in being able to influence our behaviour has not been widely recognised in psychiatry and medicine.[12] It allows a person to feel much less helpless and more in control and gives immediate and 'truthful' feedback about 'the problem'. One Oxford study has shown that people with high blood pressures who were taught to monitor their blood pressures daily showed therapeutically significant falls in blood pressure within a few weeks.

Relaxation and Breathing Control. The most direct way to reduce anxiety is to learn to alter it by directly controlling one or more of its physiological components. The most widely used technique is progressive muscle relaxation, in which the client learns an active method of relaxing her muscles and thereby reducing feelings of anxiety.[13] As with all skills, it is harder to acquire when someone is in an acute state of anxiety but it may be useful with well-preserved elderly people who have specific or less severe anxiety. An alternative method of relaxation which elderly people often find easier to use involves autogenic imagery. In this, a pleasant image, such as lying on a beach on a warm summer's day, is brought vividly to mind, producing a feeling of calm. Providing the elderly person with a pre-recorded cassette of such a scene for use at home gives her a means of controlling feelings of anxiety at any time during the day, with a minimum of extra effort. In all cases clear explanation, self-monitoring and a very gradual approach will aid the development of relaxation skills.

Another direct factor which has recently been shown to be important in the genesis and maintenance of anxiety is breathing pattern.[14] Hyperventilation which is characterised by shallow, thoracic, rapid breathing has been shown to generate unpleasant physiological symptoms within the space of a few minutes.[15] It is the author's own experience that this phenomenon occurs commonly in elderly people with anxiety. Reduction of anxiety in these cases will often depend on relearning a normal breathing pattern. This involves learning to slow the speed of breathing and use of the diaphragm rather than the upper chest. This approach remains largely untried with elderly people, perhaps because those who present with difficulties often have many years history of an abnormal breathing pattern.

Case 6.4:

Mrs I.S. was a 66-year-old with a three-year history of apparent depressive illness, and agoraphobic symptoms. On assessment she appeared to be emaciated and sat continuously overbreathing (at a rate of over 20/minute) with her breathing pattern the reverse of normal. It had been noted from the medical notes that gastroscopy had confirmed inflammation in her stomach and her stomach pain was still being treated with little success. Compliance had been equivocal on previous antidepressant treatment, so a further trial was instituted which produced no improvement and marked side effects. This lent further weight to the view that one important factor in Mrs I.S.'s state was her hyperventilation. A programme of breathing retraining was instituted. It took approximately 20 sessions for Mrs I.S. to be able to learn to take *one* in/out breath normally (using her diaphragm correctly). Unfortunately, at this time the physician treating her gastritis prescribed 5 mg Valium tds and failed to inform the GP. This completely undermined her progress, as she had to be slowly taken off this medication because of side effects, producing a worsening of her stomach pain and exacerbation of her anxiety. After 40 sessions, Mrs I.S. can now breathe normally for one to two minutes at a time, but her stomach pain continues to interfere with her breathing pattern and the anxiety resulting from hyperventilation continues to exacerbate her gastritis. Help and support continues to be given in this case although the prognosis is not good.

The earlier identification of such factors by those working both in psychiatry and general medicine could lead to improved treatment of this disorder. We in our Western culture have something to learn about preventative work from the East. In China, the basic health exercise for elderly people, Tai Chi Chuan, a slow, flowing, dance-like series of movements, involves learning to control breathing through use of the diaphragm, as well as learning to use different muscle groups simultaneously without tensing other parts of the body. Thus, this 3,000-year-old exercise embodies the principles of correct breathing and relaxation.

Interpersonal Difficulties. For convenience, the different factors affecting anxiety have been considered separately. However, most work with the elderly client is likely to involve an approach which considers all these factors and their likely interaction. As will be seen in Chapter 8, 'Individual and Family Therapy', the interpersonal context must also be considered.

Case 6.5:

Mrs F.P. was a 67-year-old divorced woman who presented with abdominal pain and anxiety. She was referred by the physician involved as physical investigations had proved negative. Her present difficulties with anxiety and abdominal pain had developed gradually when the daughter she was closest to committed suicide some three years previously. The initial interview in which she said she 90 per cent accepted that there was no serious disease present indicated that the extensive physical investigations up to this point had helped her to accept that her anxiety level was the real problem.

Table 6.2 gives a simplified view of her eight-session therapy. In this case a joint family session with her two other daughters, looking at the effect the third daughter's death had upon all of them, was the crucial factor in consolidating the progress Mrs F.P. made. The practical outcome was more involvement by the daughters and at three-month follow-up their mother was going out regularly, had resumed reading for the first time in years and was planning to go for a holiday abroad with her sister.

Table 6.2: Mrs F.P.'s Problems and Treatment Approach

Problems	Therapeutic input
Diffuse anxiety	Self-monitoring, relaxation exercises
Anxiety related to trips out	Information and support, setting gradually increasing goals
Poor sleep pattern	General information regarding sleep promotion
Stomach pain	Information regarding pain and anxiety
Social isolation, loss of confidence	Day centre arranged, as actual social skills good
Closest daughter's suicide	Bereavement work, discussing circumstances surrounding this
Remaining children not visiting enough	Family meeting held

Coping With Failure

It has been the aim throughout this chapter to present a realistic account of the challenges facing a team working with this particularly difficult group of elderly people. However, in doing this, it may be reasonably argued that we have erred on the side of being too optimistic about the prognosis of elderly people presenting with hypochondriacal complaints. This may in part be because it is difficult to present the reader with true-to-life accounts of particular patients treatment through the use of short written case-histories. Some of the 'successes' illustrated give no feeling of the high levels of personal stress experienced by the professionals involved and the reliance of those professionals on the support and empathy of the team within which they worked. It is the authors' opinion that quality of care, and indeed success in helping such people in distress, could be greatly improved if a *genuine* team approach was adopted more widely in psychiatric practice.

The optimism in this chapter perhaps also reflects our view that there is no purpose to be served by adopting a pessimistic stance when attempting to help an elderly person, whatever the problem. In fact, being pessimistic may hinder the professional's ability to continue to utilise a constructive problem-solving model. If we continue to attempt to solve the therapeutic problems we face, however difficult, then there is always some hope of success. If we stop trying to solve the problems because we do not believe they can be solved, then the outcome is inevitable — failure.

Having said this, there remains the question of how the 'front-line' professional, whether key worker or GP, copes with a family or individual who appears to undermine every effort to help, or indeed does not respond to any of the interventions made.

When seeing individuals who have been labelled as 'difficult' in their contact with other agencies, particularly if a number of family members or other carers are involved, the kind of initial interview carried out is often crucial. The simple information-gathering interview, as in Case 6.2, leading to an agreed programme of intervention within three sessions, and a successful outcome, can prove disastrous with 'difficult' cases. One possible explanation for this phenomenon is that for some individuals and their carers, direct advice is perceived as being told they have not tried, or have been 'lazy' in their efforts to change. Whilst there is little research looking at this, most clinicians will be able to recall such families, who appear extremely threatened by the simplest of advice. The family who responds to advice with 'Oh we've tried that', is giving a clear message to the advice giver that they do not feel he has listened to their problems. Herr and Weakland (1979) who looked in detail at counselling elderly people and their families have emphasised the role of the assessment interview as part of the intervention, highlighting techniques which are likely to maximise the co-operation of the family.[16] After defining the problem more clearly, moving from the global to the specific, the interview centres on looking at all the solutions 'tried' by the family and others, *including failed solutions*. Practically, such an approach allows the therapist to see what solutions have not worked, what solutions have failed because they were not properly implemented, and what solutions may be causing or exacerbating the problem. As part of this, the therapist resists offering advice in the early stages and even if it is obvious that a solution the relative has adopted is exacerbating the situation, does not state this to the family. This kind of approach was used in Case 6.4, partly because the family was noted not to have complied with previous attempts to help and the caring son as having written regular letters of complaint. Although the interventions adopted did not succeed in helping this lady, there was never any problem with compliance and the son and father were satisfied that, psychologically, all that could be done was being done.

Finally, it is noted that even with the most flexible use of such skills, there are a few elderly people with hypochondriacal complaints to whom it is impossible to give any help. In these cases it is worth remembering Figure 6.3 which indicates that any increased anxiety is likely to excaberate the hypochondriacal behaviour. Not adding to anxiety can be achieved by providing the client with a clear, *non-punitive* structure. A brief example of one such plan which might be used to try to cope with an elderly person who phones the GP's surgery ten times a week complaining of serious illnesses is shown in Table 6.3. Similar plans can be drawn up to cope with patients who hound the doctor or nurse on the ward, or who talk incessantly about their symptoms and not themselves. Providing such a clear structure may not be a cure, but helps to limit the damage patients do to themselves, opens the way to improvement and may reduce the stress felt by the professionals involved by giving them a coping strategy.

Table 6.3: Examples of a Plan for Use with Hypochondriacal Patient who Rings the GP Surgery Ten Times per Week for Home Consultations

1. One regular visit per week (not following a call). To include 20 minutes' physical examination, firm reassurance.
2. Only one named GP to provide consultations (the GP who is most willing to see the client).
3. An extra visit is carried out if two days pass without any phone call from patient (criteria to be altered if situation improves).
4. If GP has to respond to a 'false' urgent call, e.g. patient feigning heart attack, visit should be conducted in a calm manner, examination should be the minimum necessary to exclude a real medical emergency and should be time limited, i.e. five minutes or less. The GP should leave as soon as possible with a brief informative comment to patient (e.g. 'You are not suffering from a heart attack, I have to leave now, I have other patients to see').
5. GP's secretary is given precise instructions as to what information to give during phone calls by patient.

Conclusion

In this chapter the importance of psychiatric diagnosis and psychological factors in the management of hypochondriasis has been illustrated. When used correctly medical and psychological approaches are complementary rather than exclusive in nature. Neglecting one or the other is poor practice. Developing effective care for elderly people with such problems will depend on psychiatrists', psychologists' and other professional groups' acceptance of the complementary nature of their skills.

Notes

1. Schulz, R., 'Emotionality and Ageing: A Theoretical and Empirical Analysis', *Journal of Gerontology,* 37, 1982, 42–51.

2. Kenyon, F.E., 'Hypochondriasis: A Clinical Study', *British Journal of Psychiatry,* 110, 1964, 478–88.

3. Wilson, L.A., Lawson, I.R. and Brass, H. 'Multiple Disorders in the Elderly', *Lancet,* 2, 27 October, 1962, 841–3.

4. De Alarcon, R. 'Hypochondriasis and Depression in the Aged', *Gerontologia Clinica,* 6, 1964, 266–77.

5. Bradley, J.J., 'Severe Localised Pain Associated with Depressive Syndrome', *British Journal of Psychiatry,* 109, 1963, 741–5.

6. Webb, H.E. and Lascelle, R.G., 'Treatment of Facial and Head Pain Associated with Depression', *Lancet,* 1, 17 February, 1962, 355.

7. Block, A.R., Kremer, E.F. and Gaylor, M., 'Behavioural Treatment of Chronic Pain: The Spouse as a Discriminative Cue for Pain Behaviour', *Pain,* 9, 1980, 243–52.

8. Wooley, S.C., Blackwell, B. and Winget, C., 'A Learning Theory Model of Chronic Illness Behaviour. Treatment and Research', *Psychosomatic Medicine,* 40, 1978, 5, 379–401.

9. Roth, P.M., Caron, M.S., Ort, R.S., Berger, D.G., Albee, G.W. and Streeter, G.A., 'Patients' Beliefs about Peptic Ulcer and its Treatment', *Annals of Internal Medicine,* 56, 1962, 72–80.

10. Trethowan, W.H., 'Pain in the Mind', *The Midland Journal of Psychotherapy,* 1, 1983, 56–64.

11. Kellner, R. 'Psychotherapeutic Strategies in Hypochondriasis. A Clinical Study', *American Journal of Psychotherapy,* 36, 1982, 2, 146–57.

12. Kanfer, F.H., 'Self-regulation: Research Issues and Speculations' in C. Neuringer and J.L. Michael (eds), *Behaviour Modification in Clinical Psychology* (New York, Appleton Century Crofts, 1970).

13. Rimm, D.C. and Masters, J.C., *Behaviour Therapy. Techniques and Empirical Findings* (Academic Press, London, 1974).

14. Ley, R. 'Agoraphobia, the Panic Attack and the Hyperventilation Syndrome', *Behaviour Research and Therapy,* 23, 1985, 1, 79–82

15. Lum, L.C., 'The Syndrome of Habitual Hyperventilation', in O. Hill (ed.), *Modern Trends in Psychosomatic Medicine, Volume 3* (Butterworth, London, 1976).

16. Herr, J.J. and Weakland, J.H., *Counselling Elders and Their Families. Practical Techniques for Applied Gerontology* (Springer, New York, 1979).

HALLUCINATIONS AND PERSECUTORY
STATES

Hallucinations and persecutory phenomena often go hand-in-hand. When we consider the human need to make sense of a situation, this is perhaps not surprising. A person who has an inexplicable sensory experience may well find an explanation in a persecutory delusion. Despite the frequent interaction of hallucinations and persecutory states, they are not always related. For clarity, we will therefore in this chapter first deal with the interpretation of hallucinations and then consider separately persecutory phenomena.

Hallucinations

The type of hallucination is often a guide to diagnosis. Auditory hallucinations are found most commonly in schizophrenic states, although they sometimes also occur in depressive illness, when the derogatory content is consonant with the depressed mood. Hearing one's thoughts spoken out loud or hearing two voices discussing one in the third person are, provided the patient is fully conscious, often regarded as diagnostic of schizophrenia. For a fuller discussion of these and other 'first-rank' symptoms of schizophrenia, the reader is referred to Mellor.[1] Visual hallucinations, on the other hand, are generally regarded as the hallmark of organic states, especially acute confusional states. Perhaps the best known of these are the vivid visual hallucinations of alcohol withdrawal ('delirium tremens') which can occur in other drug withdrawal states.

Case 7.1:
   D.F. was an 83-year-old widow with poor eyesight living alone but near her son. She had been on Lorazepam for many years, and fell, fracturing her femur. In hospital she made a good recovery from operation, but then seemed to become depressed. her Lorazepam was stopped, and an antidepressant started. Over the next few days she became much more disturbed, and one night believed that she had wakened to see her son being dismembered. For several days she was convinced that he had in fact been murdered. A benzodiazepine was re-started, and the problems resolved though she remained apprehensive about being discharged.

This lady illustrates the complexities of medical care for old people. She may well have had her fall precipitated by poor eyesight and medication. The subsequent visual hallucination was probably related to benzodiazepine withdrawal, poor eyesight, and possibly to the anti-cholinergic effect of the antidepressant that was started. Relative sensory deprivation through poor eyesight and hearing are important contributory factors for hallucinations and paranoid states. Indeed, the relationship between poor hearing and persecutory states has long been recognised.[2] Sometimes imparied sight may produce a frightening hallucinosis without associated persecutory phenomena, the Charles-Bonnet syndrome.[3]

Case 7.2:

Karen was an 87-year-old lady who, although severely handicapped by arthritis, lived in her own back-to-back terraced house. She suffered visual hallucinations which had developed in complexity over a six-week period until she saw images of cats in her bedroom, a number seven bus going across her sitting-room ceiling and a man building a glass box in the corner. These hallucinations were of normal size and colour, became more apparent in the evening and night-time and were only in one sensory modality. Karen was intellectually completely intact on brief testing and perplexed and frightened by her experience. The psychiatrist started her on a small dose of thioridazine as symptomatic treatment and arranged further investigations. An investigation by a neurologist into the possibility of temporal lobe seizures (TLE) was negative and drew the unhelpful comment 'I imagine these are just delusions of the senile brain'. A detailed neuropsychological investigation following this showed Karen was intellectually well preserved with good insight into her condition. An EEG (electroencephalogram) was arranged but the patient refused this, mainly because of embarrassment as she was bald and wore a wig! Her hallucinatory experiences were not stereotyped and there was nothing else to suggest TLE so we concluded that this was probably a case of visual hallucinations due to sensory deprivation.

The psychologist's counselling for Karen consisted mainly of reassurance and explanation and the thioridazine was discontinued. The hallucinations continued but she did not find them so troublesome. She eventually confided that she had put off seeking help for several weeks because she was afraid she was going mad.

Other types of hallucination, e.g. tactile and olfactory, are rarer in old age. Tactile hallucinations of a sexual kind are found not infrequently in paraphrenia. The hallucination of a bad smell emanating from the patient's body is sometimes found in severe depression.

The *content* of an hallucination can also help in diagnosis. Hallucinations consistent with a poor self-image, for example, voices accusing the patient of acts of which she believes she is guilty, or hallucinations that the patient smells, linked perhaps with the delusions that she is dirty, are often associated with a severely depressed mood. Not all hallucinations in depressive illness have an obviously depressive content. Associated findings such as poor eyesight or hearing or acute physical illness can also point to the diagnosis and management. One condition in which mentally well people sometimes experience auditory or visual hallucinations is following bereavement (see Chapter 4).

The commonest cause of predominantly visual hallucination in old age is an organic brain disorder, often an acute confusional state, but sometimes a dementia, especially of the multi-infarct type. The role of medication, and drug (especially benzodiazepine) withdrawal, in precipitating confusional states must be stressed. The commonest cause of predominantly auditory hallucinations is paraphrenia, though depressive disorders and bereavement reactions also account for a proportion. Visual and hearing impairment are important in increasing an elderly person's susceptibility to hallucination regardless of diagnosis.

In temporal lobe epilepsy, stereotyped hallucinations may occur, sometimes in several modalities. Figure 7.1 provides a flow chart to assist in the diagnosis of hallucinations.

Persecutory States

We admire children for their innocence but go to great pains to teach them to be suspicious of the motives of others, first through fairy tales and then through specific warnings not to take sweets from, or go with strangers. Becasue there are unscrupulous people who will exploit or harm vulnerable children or old people, we have to encourage a certain amount of suspiciousness. Some people take this necessary caution too far, and become suspicious of all outsiders. People with such a personality often develop an isolated, self-sufficient life-style which enables them to avoid warm social contact with other people. In old age, physical or psychiatric illness suddenly puts them in a position where they do need outside help, but find this very difficult to accept. Organic brain disease

Figure 7.1: Flow Chart for the Diagnosis of Hallucinations

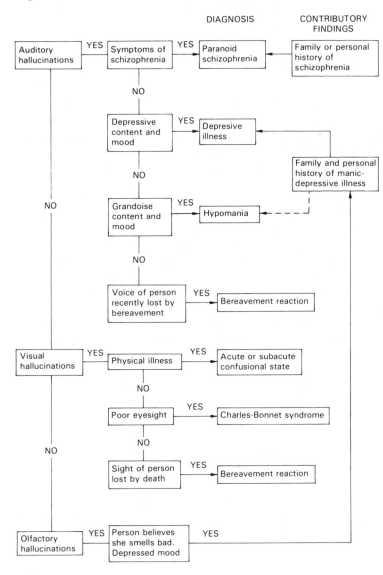

N.B.: Tactile hallucinations and other rarer hallucinations which usually, if they are present, form part of the symptoms of schizophrenia, have been omitted for simplicity. Hallucinations in one of the several modalities also occur in temporal lobe epilepsy.

may supervene either coincidentally or as a consequence of a restricted or bizarre diet. Alternatively, a frank paraphrenic illness may develop with delusions and hallucinations.

Paraphrenia

The existence of this disorder as a separate clinical entity has been called into question. It is the latest-onset form of schizophrenia and was defined operationally by Roth[4] as a late-onset disorder characterised by 'a well organised system of paranoid delusions with or without auditory hallucinations existing in the setting of a well-preserved personality and affective response. Some writers have failed to separate this disorder from organic paranoid states, but, provided that the distinction is observed, late paraphrenia is a valid diagnostic category with a characteristic natural history. The history of this diagnostic category is discussed in detail by Grahame[5] in a paper on late paraphrenia which argues firmly in favour of retaining this diagnosis. Paraphrenia develops in people, usually women, of a paranoid or schizoid premorbid personality. They are usually single, or have had unsatisfactory marriages and sexual adjustment. They have few or no surviving children, and are often chronically hard of hearing. People of lower social class seem to be more vulnerable and sufferers often live in substandard inner city housing.

First admission rates for schizophrenia peak in young adulthood but, especially for women, there seems to be a further peak in the over-75-year-old age group. This may reflect the influence of non-dementing organic brain damage, of increasing stresses as capacity for independent living is compromised by other physical or psychiatric problems or of sensory deprivation. Up to 10 per cent of elderly psychiatric inpatients suffer from paraphrenia though we do not find it so common in our inpatient practice, and the prevalence rate in the community is probably less then 1 per cent. Feelings of depressed mood are not uncommon in elderly paraphrenics although the depression is almost invariably seen by the patient as a reaction to perceived wrongs. The presence of paranoid symptoms in some patients suffering from moderate depressive illness can lead to difficulties in diagnosis. Schizoid premorbid personality is one of the best diagnosis pointers for paraphrenia whereas a personal or family history of affective disorder usually points to a depressive diagnosis.

Case 7.3:

Mrs B.K. was a 78-year-old widow who lived alone in an eighth floor high rise flat. When seen at home she was, she said, feeling depressed and thought this might be due to the attentions paid her by a man at the day centre she attended. There were no clear hallucinations or delusions but the patient seemed cognitively slowed and preoccupied. The psychiatrist thought this might be evidence of a subtly varying level of awareness and arranged admission with a provisional diagnosis of early dementia, possibly of a metabolic origin. On the ward, the patient developed a delusional conviction that another (male) patient was following her, and wanted to get into bed with her. She had auditory hallucinations of a voice telling her what to do and believed that her hands were being moved by an outside influence. The diagnosis of paraphrenia was made and she was treated successfully with Trifluoperazine. No metabolic abnormalities were detected.

Late paraphrenia responds well to treatment with neuroleptics, provided the patient can be persuaded to take them. Building a therapeutic relationship with the elderly paraphrenic person is often particularly difficult but community nurses who often give depot neuroleptic preparations to these patients can become adept. Often a compromise has to be worked out in terms of dosage such that patients' symptoms are controlled sufficiently for them to carry on with everyday life without excessive side effects and with a minimum need for anti-cholinergic anti-Parkinsonian drugs which can themselves cause confusion. When depressive features persist despite adequate neuroleptic medication, antidepressant medication or ECT can be added depending on circumstances.

Symptomatic Paranoid States

Affective Illness

Chapter 4 mentions how paranoid symptoms are not uncommon in moderately depressed old people. Post[6] has discussed the mixture of schizophrenic and affective symptoms in old age. He has also described a state of 'intermediate psychotic depression' in which paranoid phenomena are relatively common and do not always have the characteristic that the patient believes the persecution is justified.

Case 7.4:

A 72-year-old widow lived in a very poor back-to-back house with her severely obsessionally neurotic daughter. The old lady was admitted to hospital with a severe psychotic depression which was initially treated with antidepressants. When she went home to the very restrictive life imposed by the daughter (who, incidentally, refused treatment for her own condition), she relapsed rapidly and had to be re-admitted. She was so severly disabled that, on this occasion, she had to be given electro-convulsive therapy (ECT). She made a stormy recovery and for a period became quite paranoid, believing that we were experimenting on her and that we wanted to get rid of her. She eventually returned to good health and with maintenance antidepressant therapy, strong social support in the home and day hospital attendance, she has remained well for a considerable time.

This case not only illustrates the way in which paranoid symptoms may form part of the symptom-picture of a depressed patient, it also illustrates how a patient can go through stages of depression during recovery. The daughter's severe obsessional neurosis also raises the question, in this family at least, of a genetic link between depressive illness and severe obsessional phenomena. In old age psychiatry, one often has the benefit not only of an antecedent family history, but also of a family history of mental illness in the patient's children. This can be diagnostically helpful, but sometimes it seems to call into question purist views of the genetics of mental illness.

Case 7.5:

L.H. was a 75-year-old widow, admitted with an attack of hypomania following a move to an old person's home. She had a history of manic-depressive illness. On this occasion her mood was euphoric and she had slight pressure of ideas. She had ideas of reference and thought that a 'type of shock' was being imposed on her body. After treatment, she returned to independent living in a new flat. Despite day hospital support, she had six futher admissions over a two-year period. On some occasions there was an element of manipulation in her addmissions but most times there was also clear evidence of depressive illness. She also developed a severe anaemia, probably of dietary origin which responded to treatment. On one occasion she again became very suspicious, accusing us of treating her as a 'guinea pig'. Recently she has remained relatively well at home on a tricyclic antidepressant with support from a community nurse and a social worker as well as day hospital and day centre attendance.

This patient who normally had recurrent depressive illness thus had a hypomanic episode with strong paranoid features. When severe persecutory phenomena occur in depressive illness or hypomania, it is fully justified to treat them in their own right with a neuroleptic drug.

Alcoholism and Drug Dependence

An isolated auditory hallucinosis or a full-blown schizophreniform illness can develop in elderly as well as younger alcoholics. Alcohol withdrawal can give rise to a state of irritability and even delirium with an affect of terror and frank persecutory phenomena. Withdrawal from phenobarbitone or other barbiturates can give a similar picture, and it is becoming clear that sudden withdrawal from benzodiazepines can also be responsible.

Case 7.6:

Mr J.H. was a 71-year-old widower who was admitted via the casualty department with an 'acute confusional state'. Despite this, he was able to give a reasonably coherent history and his memory was only minimally impaired. About a week later he suddenly became very agitated and reported odd experiences. He believed he was working a four-on-four-off shift system and said he had to go to the graveyard. He absconded in the night to one of the other wards where he tried to drag two ladies out of bed. He had to be sedated and it was only subsequently that we found he had been abusing barbituates at home. His acute confusional state had some paranoid features and was probably due to barbiturate withdrawal.

Whenever a patient develops unexpected disturbed behaviour and persecutory symptoms within a week or so of admission, the possibility of drug or alcohol withdrawal should be carefully investigated. Withdrawal states can generally be avoided by carefully planned withdrawal, if necessary with the use of a decreasing dosage regime of a sedative, non-epileptogenic drug like chlormethiazole. Long-standing use or abuse of amphetamines can also cause a schizophreniform psychosis. Psychoses arising from drug abuse can be treated symptomatically (usually in hospital) whilst the offending drug is withdrawn

Temporal Lobe Epilepsy

Although this is not specifically a condition of old age, it is worth noting that long-standing temporal lobe epilepsy can give rise to a schizophreniform psychosis.[8]

Acute Confusional States

Drug withdrawal states are really a special form of delirium or acute confusional state. Other acute confusional states have many causes (see Chapter 5). Fragmentary persecutory ideas and visual and auditory hallucinations may occur and the perplexed patient may react violently to those trying to help him. Nursing in a well-lighted environment with a regular nurse with the patient as much of the time as possible will help. Continuing reassurance and re-orientation to take account of the patient's temporarily impaired mood and memory should be offered and will do a great deal to improve the patient's co-operativeness with essential physical treatment. Occasionally, neuroleptic treatment may be justified, though, if there is a serious risk of provoking epileptic fits, a non-epileptogenic sedative such as chlormethiazole may be preferred.

Dementia

Transient persecutory phenomena, particularly accusations that mislaid objects have been stolen, are a common part of early dementia. They do not usually merit treatment in their own right. Sometimes, especially in vulnerable personalities, the paranoid symptoms may cause serious embarrassment to friends, neighbours or helping services. In these cases, symptomatic treatment with a neuroleptic such as thioridazine is justified and will often produce improvement. Very occasionally a depot neuroleptic may be needed but the dose must be kept very small in view of the increased risk of accumulation and extrapyramidal side effects.

Case 7.7:

S.C. was a 68-year-old widow who was estranged from her stepchildren. She had been married three times. She divorced her first husband, her second died suddenly and she was separated from her third. She developed the delusional belief that her third husband was coming into her flat secretly and moving furniture around. She suspected her neighbour of complicity in these plots. She had auditory hallucinations of her dead husband saying her name and believed she was 'clairvoyant'. She had minimal cognitive impairment (9/10 on the Hodkinson Memory/Information Scale) and the initial diagnosis was of paraphrenia. She was managed on neuroleptics as an inpatient initially, then as a day patient. She was also found to have a cryptogenic fibrosing alveolitis (a lung condition). She was admitted to a medical ward following a collapse with a presumptive diagnosis of stroke: her paranoid ideas had abated but she appeared confused and her memory was impaired (6/10 on the Hodkinson Memory/Information Scale). After gradual improvement she returned home but six

Figure 7.2: Flow Chart for the Diagnosis of Persecutory States

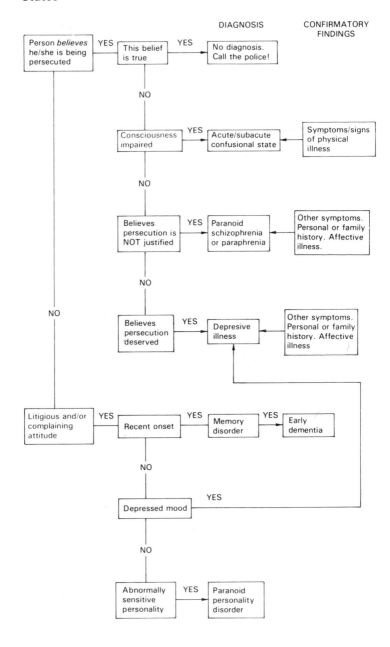

months later was readmitted with confusion and depressed mood. She was also said to be stripping off and going naked in her flat and to be neglecting herself. Her paranoid symptoms had disappeared but, in addition to slightly increased memory problems, she also had marked visuo-spatial dysfunction and neuropsychological evaluation revealed clear evidence of organic involvement. All neuroleptics were stopped without recurrence of her paranoid symptoms or improvement in her cognitive state. After another period of day hospital care she finally consented to go into residential care. She likes this and has settled well. What initially appeared to be a paraphrenic illness was thus probably a paranoid reaction to memory problems associated with early multi-infarct dementia although the possibility that she suffered from two distinct but coinicidental psychiatric disorders cannot be ruled out.

This case illustrates how difficult diagnosis can sometimes be and how helpful it can be to a patient to have a specialist service involved in management over a protracted period of time.

Figure 7.2 is a flow chart which summarises the main differential diagnosis of paranoid phenomena.

Management

Prevention

Sensory impairment and social isolation are important in all types of persistent persecutory states of late life. Deafness is usually longstanding and early detection and prescription of aids may be helpful. On the other hand, many paranoid elderly people deliberately turn off their hearing aids to limit contact with the outside world so that efforts in this direction may sometimes be unrewarding. Social isolation may even have a protective effect against the development of frank paranoid symptoms. If nothing can be done to sucessfully reduce social isolation, isolation should at least be seen as a risk factor and health and social services should keep a particularly close, though unobtrusive, watch on this vulnerable group. If simple isolation seems to be developing into frank paranoid illness, then sympathetic but firm early intervention is called for.

A Personal Approach

An accurate diagnosis is essential and this discussion presupposes that any medically treatable condition such as paraphrenia or physical illness has been diagnosed and treated. The major task for the therapeutic team is often to persuade the patient to accept such needed intervention. If a specialist opinion is called for, whenever possible the specialist should be introduced to the patient by a person with whom the patient has a reasonable relationship (often the social worker or general practitioner). A key worker should be appointed as early as possible in the management of the case. It will be this person's task to win the confidence of the old person as far as possible. An understanding approach which respects the patient's need for social distance often works best. If memory is impaired, the patient may well still remember the visitor's face and whether its last appearance was pleasant or unpleasant! The first few contacts with the key worker should be used for getting to know the patient rather than persuading her to accept a particular line of treatment or to come into hospital. If hospital admission is essential for an unwilling patient (e.g. in the acutely disturbed paraphrenic patient), then this should be organised by the general practitioner and the specialist who made the assessment visit using compulsory powers if necessary. The key worker should be kept out of this if possible. Some strategies for dealing with confused talk, taken from a book on reality orientation,[9] are summarised in Table 7.1.

Table 7.1: Strategies for Dealing with Confused Talk

1.	Tactfully disagree (on less sensitive subjects), or
2.	Change the subject — discuss something more concrete, or
3.	Acknowledge the feelings expressed — ignore the content

Source: Holden and Woods (1982).[9]

These strategies are relevant whether the patient is confused or not. One should avoid confirming delusions ('for the sake of a quiet life') but one should also avoid confrontation over delusions which will only lead to further entrenchment. Above all, one should always be scrupulously honest and open with paranoid patients. They will usually respect the doctor who says he is going to insist they come into hosptial far more than the one who disappears only to be followed a few hours later by others arriving to arrange a compulsory admission.

Medication

Fortunately, most hallucinatory and paranoid states show some response to neuroleptic medication. Where there is organic brain disease, however, the balance between the anti-psychotic effects of the drugs and unwanted side effects if often difficult to achieve. Neuroleptic drugs are often cumulative in old age, and dosage regimes need to be monitored and often changed. Generally, one aims to keep the dose of the neuroleptic as low as possible rather than introducing anti-cholinergic anti-Parkinsonian drugs which may themselves precipitate confusion. Drug treatment is discussed further in Chapter 10.

Conclusion

Paranoid or persecutory phenomena are found in old-age mental illness of all types, often in association with sensory deprivation. They are most consistently found in developed form in the late-onset form of schizophrenia, late paraphrenia, for which specific medical treatment is available. Whatever the underlying cause of persecutory phenomena, the health care professionals' approach and ability to build workable relationships with a very difficult group of patients is cardinal to successful treatment.

Notes

1. Mellor, C.S., 'First Rank Symptoms of Schizophrenia', *British Journal of Psychiatry,* 117, 1970, 15–23.

2. Cooper, A.F., Curry, A.R., Kay, D.W.K., Garside, K.F. and Roth, M., 'Hearing Loss in Paranoid and Affective Psychoses of the Elderly', *Lancet,* 1974, 2, 851–4.

3. Berrios, C.F. and Brook, P. 'Visual Hallucinations and Sensory Delusions in the Elderly', *British Journal of Psychiatry,* 144, 1984, 662–4.

4. Roth, M., 'The Natural History of Mental Disorder in Old Age', *Journal of Mental Science,* 101, 1955, 281–301.

5. Grahame, P., 'Late Paraphrenia', *British Journal of Hospital Medicine,* 27, 1982, 522–8.

6. Post, F., 'Schizoaffective Symptomatology in Late Life', *British Journal of Psychiatry,* 118, 1971, 437–45.

7. Post, F., 'The Management and Nature of Depressive Illness in Late Life: A Follow Through Study, *British Journal of Psychiatry,* 121, 1972, 393–404.

8. Slater, E., 'The Schizophrenia-like Psychoses of Epilepsy in *Current Problems in Neuropsychiatry,* (Royal Medico-Psychological Assocation, London, 1969).

9. Holden, U.P. and Woods, R.T., *Reality Orientation: Psychological Approaches to the 'Confused' Elderly,* (Churchill Livingstone, London, 1982).

8 INDIVIDUAL AND FAMILY THERAPY

Individual Therapy

Most people at some time in their lives have psychological problems of one kind or another, yet continue to lead satisfying and fulfilled lives. They either learn to cope with their problems or gain sufficient support and help from their personal relationships to overcome them. For a few, however, the level of distress becomes so great that their ability to cope with everyday life becomes seriously undermined. Elderly people are more vulnerable to psychological problems than most, as they have to face many changes in a short period of time. Not only must they cope with their failing physical functions, but they must also adapt to a wide variety of changes, such as loss of earning power, old friends and status. Given this, most elderly people present a remarkable picture of adjustment.

Rather than viewing those distressed elderly people who come for help as having deeply flawed personalities, we prefer to view them as having either failed to use the right strategies, or as lacking the appropriate support, to deal with their problems. We believe that the application of psychological principles, especially learning principles, can be effective in changing maladaptive, unwanted, or distressing thoughts, feelings and behaviour. Individual psychological therapy is the approach of choice when an individual is cognitively well preserved, where the problem does not seem to be directly related to the reaction of family members or relatives and where the person, to some extent, is ready to accept the psychological nature of her distressing experiences rather than, for example, seeing these purely in physical terms.

It should be clear from these opening comments that the present authors believe that the view which has often been presented, of elderly people being inappropriate candidates for individual psychological therapy, is both ill informed and illogical. This feeling of pessimism seems to have arisen because the psychological consequences of ageing were seen as arising out of a biological process which was by and large irreversible. In fact, the consistent effect of ageing is to make an individual's behaviour more dependent on the environment in its broadest sense. Thus, rather than making the actions of the therapist irrelevant, ageing makes them more important in determining the probability of completing a successful therapeutic intervention. Individual therapy with elderly people thus requires all the skills and techniques which may be used with younger people, but also additional skills to take account of the specific effects of ageing in the individual.

Whatever the client's age, the first step in individual therapy is to develop a therapeutic relationship, as this is necessary for her active co-operation in the use of therapeutic techniques, and may also produce change of itself.[1] This can be fostered in a number of ways. The therapist should be non-judgemental, accepting the client as a valued individual regardless of her behaviour, thoughts or feelings (without making moral judgements). He should make active attempts to understand what the client has experienced by regularly rephrasing and summarising what she says in the interview, giving her an opportunity to correct him if necessary. Also, an active concern for the client's needs should be shown within the session, for example responding with warmth, acceptance and comfort, if she becomes distressed.

A consistent view which has emerged from reports of work with elderly people, has been the importance of the therapist taking the role of an active advocate for the client, rather than being neutral.[2] Age brings with it an increasing likelihood of physical infirmity and illness. Lungs and circulatory systems decrease in efficiency and muscles tend to waste, making it harder to do the constructive things that every younger person takes for granted; in particular it becomes harder to translate new or revived goals from ideas into action. Not only is this the case because it requires more physical effort, but because the increasing awareness of reducing capacity inevitably leads to a greater degree of conservatism. Greater difficulties in the generalisation of behaviour to the client's natural environment must be anticipated with elderly people. The therapist as an active and helpful ally can help to overcome these difficulties and it is likely that successful therapy with elderly people requires an even greater emphasis on the involvement of other staff, for example in a day hospital setting. Changes facilitated in therapy can be encouraged by the staff and consolidated outside therapy. As part of this active role the therapist should always arrange to hold the initial assessment interview in the elderly person's home. Too often the sheer physical obstacle of having to travel two or three miles to a hospital's outpatients department overcomes the elderly person's wish to receive therapeutic help. Not only can a visit to her home increase compliance, but the therapist can also get a clearer idea of how each individual copes in her own territory and can assess the degree to which social and environmental factors may be contributing to her difficulties.

Ageing, Cognitive Function and Therapy

Early research not only consistently over-estimated the changes in cognitive ability found in older people but also regarded these changes as deficits. The difficulties in appropriately interpreting research in this area can be illustrated by referring to one reported study which compared a group of college students with a group of young children (aged five to six years).[3] Both groups were asked to attempt to predict which of three lights would come on next, over a number of trials. Unknown to the participants, it was arranged that light 1 would come on 60 per cent of the time, light 2 would come on 30 per cent of the time and light 3 10 per cent of the time. It was found that the young children performed consistently more successfully than the college students on this task. Such findings illustrate the dangers of viewing cognitive development as a move towards perfection, as any change in cognitive ability will lead to both benefits and costs depending on the situation and the task involved. Bearing this in mind, there are some changes in cognitive function occuring with ageing which do have direct implications for therapy.

Abstract Ability. Changes in this area have been most dramatically illustrated by Walker (1982) who found that the failure rate on a test of ability to shift set (measured by the person's ability to classify groups of objects on different dimensions such as colour and shape) rose from 10 per cent in those aged 60 to 64 years to 92 per cent in those over 80 years of age.[4] This result suggests a substantial decrease in at least one aspect of abstract ability between 60 and 80 years of age. Such changes in ability may cause difficulties when the therapist fails to show the client that he has a good understanding of the personal meaning of her psychological problems, as can happen when the psychiatric interview is insensitive, or the client's behaviour is explained using esoteric or technical language. A more general implication arising from this study is that not only do elderly people have special needs as compared with younger people but that the over 60 or 65 population is not necessarily homogeneous. This reaffirms the importance of assessing the individual elderly person's needs and assets before carrying out a therapeutic intervention.

Semantic Memory and Information Processing. Experimental studies have been carried out comparing the ability of normal younger people, as compared to normal elderly people, to detect changes in a spoken text.[5] Although both groups were found to be broadly equivalent in their ability to detect non-semantic changes in the text (i.e. changes not affecting the meaning), the ability to detect semantic change (i.e. alterations in the meaning) was markedly worse amongst the elderly subjects, after a delay. The implications for therapy are clear, that older people may be disadvantaged in recalling the meaning being 'given' to them by the therapist. Although the experimental situations used were different and considerably harder than normal conversation (where, for example, information is more related to the situational context), it might be suggested that as the therapy becomes more verbal and interpretive in nature (as in traditional psychoanalysis) the elderly client will have increasing difficulty. Interestingly, elderly subjects in another study initially given a written passage and unlimited time did not show this effect.[6] This indicates that a therapist should carefully pace the introduction of new information, and whenever possible attempt to reduce any handicap by carefully structuring the session and writing down any didactic information to be remembered. Research has shown that the average younger person will forget at least one-half of the verbal instructions given by a GP within five minutes of leaving the surgery. Ley (1977) has made several specific suggestions for increasing the amount of information patients are likely to recall (see Table 8.1).[7] The appropriate presentation of information to the elderly person is likely to be even more important.

Table 8.1: Suggestions for Increasing Amount and Content of Patients' Recall

1.	Whenever possible, provide patients with instructions and advice at the start of the information to be presented.
2.	When providing patients with instructions and advice, stress how important they are.
3.	Use short words and short sentences.
4.	Use explicit categorisation where possible.
5.	Repeat things where feasible.
6.	When giving advice make it as specific, detailed and concrete as possible.

Case 8.1:

Mr H.R. was a 65-year-old man who had a twelve-year history of depression. He had always been a perfectionist about his work and had coped well until the combination of a mild heart attack and the side effects of medication led to increasing stress at work. He continued working, but the burden became intolerable, and following a number of periods of 'illness' he received an acrimonious early retirement. He also developed secondary erectile impotence during this period. His problems and the methods used to tackle them are summarised in Table 8.2.

Table 8.2: Mr H.R.'s Problems and Treatment Methods

Problem	Therapeutic approach	Therapy involves
Depressed mood	Cognitive therapy	Identify thoughts triggering low mood. Develop more realistic thoughts
Intrusive disturbing images from recent past about all the things he should have done at work (but didn't)	Bereavement model	Allow time to talk about and re-evaluate past events. Allow the expression of distress (crying)
Anxiety	Education and anxiety management	Provide explanatory model, teach self-monitoring of anxiety level, use of relaxation and systematic desensitisation
Decrease in erectile ability	Not seen as problem by Mr and Mrs H.R. Assessed as not relevant to other difficulties	Support their perceptions, positively view their adaptation to their change in sexual response

Following a detailed assessment interview, the contract of ten sessions was agreed upon. Towards the end of ten sessions, Mr H.R. was beginning to identify the unrealistic thoughts which had triggered his periods of depression and began to develop more realistic thoughts. It also became apparent that he suffered considerable anxiety at various times during the day and his initial attempts at controlling this proved fairly successful. He began to be able to control the intrusive disturbing images from his recent past and these became less distressing. A further ten sessions of therapy were agreed upon. His progress continued and he was successfully weaned off his antidepressant medication at the third attempt, the previous attempt having failed because of the anxiety.

Mr H.R. is reasonably confident about the future, feeling much more in control of his anxiety and much less troubled by incidents from the past.

Case 8.2:

Mr G.S. was a 66-year-old man who three months before the referral had completed his third spell in prison. He had served three years for homosexual activity and mutual masturbation with boys under the age of consent. His previous history was long and complicated, but it was noted that he had first experienced orgasm at the age of about 13 when he was involved in mutual masturbation with a boy of a similar age. Mutual masturbation with similar aged boys continued to be his only sexual outlet until he reached his mid-twenties.

He had been married twice: The first marriage had been reasonably successful until his wife died from a bowel complaint, but the second was disastrous as he had been seeking solace rather than a full relationship. His problems and the means used to tackle them are summarised in Table 8.3. Mr G.S. was accepted for treatment because he was well motivated and wanted help. Before covert sensitisation was used, Mr G.S. would feel tempted to involve himself in homosexual activity with under-aged boys about three times a week. After two sessions he had completely lost this urge and had also stopped fantasising and dreaming about such activities. The development of a sexual response to adult females proved less successful.

Table 8.3: Mr G.S.'s Problems and Treatment Methods

Problem	Therapeutic approach	Therapy involves
Illegal sexual behaviour and related fantasy and dreaming	Covert sensitisation	Associating images of illegal sexual behaviour with highly unpleasant consequences
No sexual response to adult females	Orgasmic reconditioning	Associating stimulation and ejaculation with 'normal' fantasy
No constructive life. Lots of free time	Support and problem-solving	Looking at and encouraging possible interests
Anger and shame related to previous events	Empathy and re-evaluation of events	Allowing expression of feelings and helping to re-evaluate them

There is a much higher risk of relapse in covert sensitisation if the unwanted and disturbing behaviour, when it has been removed, is not replaced by some more constructive activity which builds self-esteem and reduces the amount of purposeless time during the day. Because Mr G.S. had not really achieved a more normal sexual response it was even more important for him to develop interests during the day. He worked on this gradually and at six months' follow-up was free from these unwanted sexual urges, and actively participating in voluntary work.

Case 8.3:

As with all treatment approaches, some people do not respond to psychological therapy. Mrs T.N. was a 70-year-old widow who lived in a multi-storey block of flats. She appeared to have developed an agoraphobic syndrome 35 years previously after some years of marriage. She had a history of one hospital admission twelve years previously when she became depressed following the death of her husband. The assessment interview showed quite clearly that she had an unresolved bereavement reaction and that she still suffered from generalised anxiety.

Despite the use of a number of therapeutic approaches (Table 8.4), Mrs T.N. made no permanent progress and a supportive role was adopted. However, by gradually removing possibly damaging medication and using phenelzine (Nardil) and organising a regular home help, some stability in her situation was achieved. However, over the next year a pattern of abuse of the phenelzine emerged and a failure in the home help service to provide a consistent home help, who could build up a relationship with Mrs T.N., culminated in her emergency admission with a depressive illness. Despite her response to ECT Mrs T.N. continues to be difficult to support adequately in the community and her future remains uncertain. Recently the combination of day hospital, and a carefully regulated social network and a closely controlled dose of phenelzine has enabled Mrs T.N. to cope better than she has for many years.

Table 8.4: Mrs T.N.'s Problems and Treatment Methods

Problem	Therapeutic approach	Therapy involves
Generalised anxiety. Recurrent images of husband. Anniversary reaction.	Bereavement model	Focus on loss repeatedly until associated emotion gradually decreased
Agoraphobic anxiety	Graduated *in vivo* exposure	Gradually set increasing goals regarding distance walked
Loneliness	Problem-solving	Look at ways to help reduce feelings of loneliness

The Therapy Contract

The overall process involves a number of stages (Figure 8.1). Following a detailed assessment interview, therapist and client come to an agreement about various aspects of the proposed therapy: they agree the therapy contract. Generally, the therapy contract is time limited with a fixed number of sessions, for example, ten sessions. This is important for clients of all ages because they come to expect some benefit within a short period of time, and are thus provided with the incentive to work on their problems. With elderly people, particular care must be taken in setting goals. It should be remembered that a person with only 10 or 15 years left to live may have priorities quite different from those of a younger person. Given also that elderly people are often not allowed to choose or decide for themselves, the therapist must be very careful not to set unrealistic or unwanted goals. This was illustrated clearly in Case 8.1. Mr H.R. and his wife saw his fairly frequent erectile failure on intercourse in terms of ageing and accepted it. If an over-enthusiastic therapist had pushed them towards sex therapy, not only would their expressed needs have been ignored, but it might also have been harmful.

Figure 8.1: The Therapy Contract: A Clear Agreement is Essential when Working with Elderly People

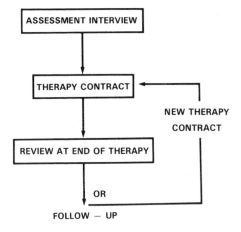

Elderly people do not necessarily find in easier to accept help from an older person, but there is certainly a danger that a younger therapist will find it harder to help the client decide on appropriate goals, or to suggest goals which the client might not have thought possible. There is no easy answer to this problem, one solution may lie in the undertaking of appropriate training. One way in which prejudice and lack of understanding of a particular group of people's needs can be reduced is by personal contact. The use of a broader therapeutic approach such as reminiscence, which fosters constructive interaction between the younger facilitator and a small group of elderly people, might help the trainee therapist develop a more sensitive awareness of appropriate goal setting within individual therapy.

Psychological Therapy

A simple way of conceptualising psychological therapy is represented in Figure 8.2 which shows the inter-dependence of a person's behaviour (what she is doing), her cognitions (what she interprets as happening) and her feelings or emotions in any situation. Psychological therapy aims at changing one or more element of this triad, leaving the person better able to cope with her own life circumstances.

Figure 8.2: Psychological Therapy: The Interactive Triad

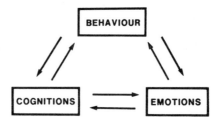

The interdependence of behaviour, cognitions and feelings can be illustrated by reference to Case 8.1. Mr H.R. was taught to understand anxiety and learned deep muscle relaxation - a direct method of reducing his level of anxiety. By changing his behaviour, learning to relax at specific times during the day, he could produce a change in his feelings and a reduction in his anxiety. When he started to perceive this control he was able to stop saying things to himself like 'I'm going mad', 'I can't cope' and instead say 'I'm starting to feel anxious again - I must do my relaxation', thus short-circuiting a vicious circle of ever-increasing anxiety. It can be seen that changing one of the components in Figure 8.2 produces feedback effects on the other two.

Common Client Issues

Certain issues are more immediately relevant to all elderly people than to most younger people. The most important of these is death. A National Institute of Mental Health sample of healthy elderly people found whilst 55 per cent showed a realistic judgement or resolution to death, 30 per cent showed overt fear and 15 per cent denial.[8] Although techniques such as systematic desensitisation and thought-stopping have been suggested as a means of reducing the fear of death in elderly clients, there is no evidence as to their effectiveness. In the absence of such evidence, the therapist must adopt a sensitive and flexible approach giving information clearly, and gently help the individual face her fears through discussion. If the old person has religious faith, it may be possible to encourage the use of this to cope with such fears.

Elderly people are not only faced with the immediacy of their own death, but have to come to terms with the death of most of their generation; close friends and relatives. The identification of a bereavement reaction contributing to a recurring psychiatric condition such as depression is not always as easy as might be expected. Those individuals who have the greatest difficulty are often most 'skilful' at avoiding their loss. They change the subject in conversation or push thoughts away from their mind whenever these bring feelings of distress to the surface. The failure to let themselves experience these intense and unpleasant emotions regularly and over extended periods of time prevents these emotions from lessening and the bereavement reaction from being eventually resolved.[9]

Case 8.4:

Mrs F.S. was a 66-year-old woman who gradually developed a depressive illness including marked obsessional checking behaviour. As she responded to antidepressant medication the community nurse involved requested psychological advice regarding her obsessional behaviour. The psychologist's assessment identified a further problem to be that of an unresolved bereavement reaction regarding the death of her husband four years previously. A programme regarding the obsessional behaviour and bereavement counselling was apparently successfully completed by the community nurse. Since the community nurse was leaving to obtain further training, the clinical psychologist agreed to carry out a follow-up. At one month follow-up it was found that Mrs F.S. was experiencing 'panics' once or twice weekly within the home and an anxiety management plan was instituted. However, it soon became apparent that she was becoming depressed again (the antidepressants having been discontinued). Although she intitially denied there was anything to make her depressed, careful questioning elicited the fact that she regularly had thoughts about her dead husband, but tended to push them out of her mind because they upset her. She also found it impossible to get out a picture of her husband, which she had put away because it upset her. Clearly, despite the community

nurse's efforts, her bereavement was still unresolved. It was agreed
with the GP to reinstitute antidepressant medication to prevent her
from becoming more depressed and a series of bereavement treatment
sessions was instituted. It was found in this case that just talking about
the husband and his death did not necessarily elicit any apparent upset
or emotion. It was only through the use of specific objects she was
avoiding such as the husband's photograph and by asking her to
visualise disturbing personal scenes, such as her husband dying in
her arms that she was able to experience the distressing emotions of
bereavement. Using this approach, the emotions gradually lessened
and although the sessions themselves were extremely stressful for both
herself and the therapist, she was always able to experience a feeling
of relief by the end of the session. It is hoped that when the bereavement is fully resolved, the risk of future episodes of depression will
have been reduced.

This example shows that those who work with elderly people must
develop the skills of bereavement counselling. As will be illustrated later
(see Case 8.7), it is important to consider a person's bereavement in
the context of other problems which may have arisen.[10]

The four cases presented illustrate the 'common-sense' approach to
psychological problems in intellectually intact old people based on a
logical appraisal of problems and the use of appropriate techniques, some
specialised and some relatively simple, to tackle problems.

Family Therapy

The importance of what others do or do not do, in relation to an elderly
person's psychological well-being has been a central theme running
through this book. Most elderly people live either with a spouse or other
relative and even those who live alone often have some contact with
relatives who are within easy travelling distance. With many elderly
people, the understanding of the family context may be the key to finding the most appropriate psychological approach. As elderly people get
older they are forced, for a variety of reasons, to become more dependent on other members of their family. This dependence makes them
more vulnerable to any changes in the family system. Widely different
approaches are used by different family therapists, and only a few have
addressed themselves specifically to how best family therapy can be

carried out with an elderly person.[11,12]

Rather than providing a particular conceptual model of family therapy, the aim in this section is to alert readers to basic good practice when working with elderly people and their families and to illustrate some commonly used concepts. The final case-history (8.7) shows how necessity may demand that the therapist change a basic practice, such as seeing the family together, to be able to carry out a successful intervention. It should also be noted that even where two different approaches are used, concepts such as the interactional system may be used in both.

The Interactional System

The focus of assessment is the family system and the interactions of its different members. Thus the involvement of the other members of the family in perpetuating the distressed or disturbing behaviour of the elderly referred patient is emphasised.

This can be illustrated by considering a family in which the father and mother lived together and their only daughter visited regularly. Before any problems emerged the father was in a full-time job approaching retirement, the mother was a conscientious housewife and the daughter visited every day to spend time with her. All were used to their particular roles and related to each other in ways which promoted mutual psychological well-being. However, the husband then retired and spent an extra eight hours a day at home. He tried to transfer his skills for organising to the home, thus usurping a role which his wife had seen as her own. This led to heated arguments between husband and wife, and the daughter, who saw this as interference by her father, sided with her mother. Thus the father, who had lost the status and self-esteem he had at work, now also faced hositility from his daughter and wife, and lapsed into depression and hostility. The system was balanced in a new way, dependent on the husband's 'illness'. Treating the old man's depression with medication was not sufficient to make him well. The family system had to be explored and altered so that he had a role which did not antagonise his wife and yet enabled him to regain his self-esteem.

Faulty Problem-solving

In our clinical experience most family members are caring and attempt to help the referred person, even when these family members appear difficult, intransigent or, occasionally, openly destructive. In general, the family members have attempted to solve problems which have arisen from a change in life circumstance in one or more family members. It is when these attempts at problem-solving are faulty that the initial problems can be exacerbated, leading eventually to the elderly family member being referred for psychiatric help.

In the previous example, it can be seen that initially the father made an attempt to solve his own problems, i.e. finding a new role which would maintain his self-esteem and use up the extra eight hours in the day. The daughter's response to this was also an attempt to solve a problem; that of the arguments between her father and mother. Unfortunately, her problem-solving attempts were faulty and led to a change in the system which resulted in her father becoming more depressed and apathetic.

Setting the Scene for Family Therapy

The initial contact between therapist and family and how this is organised is an important factor in making interventions successful. One of the most important initial tasks is to make it clear that the therapists and indeed the whole team see all the family members as having some responsibility for the referred patient's difficulties. Two rules are generally followed to encourage this idea. First, the elderly patient, who has often had a short admission, is not seen with the family until immediately after discharge. Second, in making an appointment to see the family, a carefully worded letter is sent to each of the family members including the patient in hospital. This states quite simply that the therapists consider all family members have a part to play, thus placing the responsibility squarely on the whole family rather than just on one person.

Information Gathering

It is often advisable, especially where the therapists are less experienced in working with families, that two co-therapists work together. This has a number of advantages. Large amounts of information coming from a variety of different family members can be difficult for one therapist to follow effectively. If both sexes are represented on the co-therapist's team, they may get much more information from the family.

A further problem in carrying out family therapy can be the powerful way in which family members present their view of the situation. For example, they may see the patient as mentally ill and believe they have no part to play in her well-being. Two therapists are more likely to meet such situations constructively.

As in all psychological therapy the gathering of information from a number of sources is important. Where a member of the family has been an inpatient, staff reports of the interactions between the relatives and the patient can provide useful information about how the family works. The GP, through his contact and longer-term knowledge of the family, can provide invaluable background information.

In initial interview sessions with the whole family present, therapists are interested not only in what is being said and how it is said, but also in the non-verbal communication within the family. Let us consider a particular family:

Case 8.5:

This family consisted of two sisters aged 70 and 71 living together. One who had been admitted to hospital when she was mute and unco-operative, had just been discharged. The other sister was due to be discharged from hospital following a cataract operation. Both sisters were visited regularly by their brother and sister-in-law. The initial session involved the sister who had just been discharged, her brother and sister-in-law. The sister-in-law sat next to the sister clutching at the sister's dress and patting her knee as if she were a child, whilst stridently talking across her to the therapist. The brother complained the sister was as ill as ever and still mute. When the therapist insisted that the sister-in-law address her questions to the 'mute' sister she protested vigorously and had to be repeatedly directed to do this. Even when she did direct a question to her sister, she never waited for a reply, often answering the question herself as soon as she had asked it! Interestingly, her husband had a pronounced stammer and even he had difficulty getting a word in edgeways. By the end of the session the 'mute' sister had begun to talk and, although this was only the beginning of a complicated family therapy case, a great deal of information had been gathered.

Therapeutic Strategies

A case of a mother and daughter living together illustrates two important aspects of communication in a family therapy.

Case 8.6:

Following a referral from her GP, Mrs M.M., a 70-year-old widow, was admitted with a possible depressive illness. While on the ward, she was started on antidepressant medication, although the severity of her depression was in some doubt. On her discharge, her daughter, Ms B.M., expressed considerable concern about how her mother would cope. Shortly after, the daughter made 'desperate' contact with her two GP's and the ward staff, eventually bringing her mother back two days early to see 'anybody', the daughter's response being out of all proportion to what was known of the mother's state. The conflicting advice Ms B.M. was managing to get from different members of the team effectively prevented the assigned therapists from making any progress. The situation only improved after a team meeting (a rather heated one!) in which the therapists reached an agreement with other members of the team that the daughter should be channelled in their direction.

It can be seen from this case that problems in appropriate communication with a family can be reflected outside a family. GPs and social workers are often the most vulnerable in this respect and it is important, when they know some family work is being done, that they listen sympathetically, but do not feel obliged to give advice beyond asking the family to contact their therapist.

Another important aspect of communication in family therapy is how the therapists communicate to the family members the ways in which they might need to change. The family or its individual members should never be criticised or blamed in any way. Rather, the therapist should first of all clearly acknowledge the efforts various family members have made to help each other. This is sometimes called positive connotation. Small suggestions can be made to various family members about changing what they do 'just a little bit'. Saying 'you are doing that all wrong', 'that's no good at all', 'do it this way' is unlikely to evoke a positive response. Saying 'well, that's really good, I think you put an enormous amount of effort into that, but this may need just a little change' is more likely to be favourably received. One way of acknowledging the efforts the family have made is to assess in detail what solutions the family (and other agencies) have tried and failed. This also provides the therapist with clues about what solutions may help the family, and allows the therapist to assess how well previous solutions have been implemented.

In the case described above, positive connotation proved important in helping both mother and daughter to accept and act upon the therapist's advice. As therapy progressed, it became clear that the mother's depression was a reaction to her daughter's bouts of excessive drinking and disastrous adventures with men. A vicious downward spiral of her daughter's drinking worsening mother's depression, leading to more drinking by the daughter, was interrupted by the therapy. This family dyad remains vulnerable as both are dependent on each other with few outside interests or social contacts. Because of this, the only rational psychological intervention is one which considers them both.

Whilst it is generally regarded as more desirable to see the family together, it is shown elsewhere in this book (see Case 6.2 and 9.5) that on occasion it may be necessary and indeed more effective to intervene with a key member of the family. The case presented next is the treatment of a family problem in which the family could not be seen together because of the wishes of the referred client.

Case 8.7:

Mrs K.R. was a 68-year-old widow who lived by herself in a well-kept semi-detached house, with a kitchen overflowing with plants and flowers. She had four married children living in the same city and had worked throughout her life until she had to nurse her husband till his death some three and a half years ago. On meeting her it was clear that she felt her central problem was lack of input she got from her children since her husband's death. When this emerged, the possibility of arranging a family meeting was generally discussed, but she did not want this, partly because of her fear of upsetting them. She had also not told her family that she was visiting a psychologist. A summary of the treatment methods used with Mrs K.R. are presented in Table 8.5. In the second session after the assessment interview, the issues surrounding her family's 'neglect' became clearer, when she revealed the last words uttered by her husband before his death which were 'who will look after you when I'm gone because your children won't'. This had played on her mind because she had been unable to share it with anyone (especially not her family) and indeed one daughter refused ever to visit the house again, because it reminded her of her father! Following this, it was possible to explore the implications of her own behaviour, not being appropriately assertive for fear of losing the remaining love of her children, on the kind of input she wanted to get from her family.

Interestingly, during the third session she reported having destroyed some old tablets she had been keeping to kill herself with. This emphasises the importance that a good therapeutic relationship can have prior to any more direct intervention. This case also illustrates the importance of considering non-psychological factors in the maintenance of problems such as anxiety and sleeplessness, which she reported. To cope with an empty day Mrs K.R. would make regular pots of tea and it was calculated that she was drinking about 40 cups per day. She was quite willing to cut her intake when the stimulant effects of tea were explained.

Table 8.5: Mrs K.R.'s Problems and Treatment Methods

Problem	Therapeutic approach	Therapy involves
Unhappiness with extent of children's involvement	Family meeting refused Reattribution model and assertive skills	Re-evaluating her influence on her children's behaviour towards her, emphasising ways she might change things, by changing her own behaviour
Husband's death and circumstances surrounding	Bereavement and reattribution model	Reducing her avoidance of situations which evoke his memory, and sharing and re-evaluating the circumstances of his death
Headache and general anxiety	Anxiety management and cognitive therapy	Refused relaxation, so educational approach adopted which showed links between her unhappy thoughts and her headaches
Tea over-indulgence (40 cups/day)	Simple education and advice	Advice and explanation with alternative drinks discussed

Conclusion

It has been one aim of this chapter to illustrate the flexibility with which psychological interventions need to be made. Such interventions should be a response to the circumstances of each individual family. This last example shows quite clearly that the dividing line between individual and family therapy is not as sharp as it sometimes seems. However, therapists need to be clear about the kind of intervention they are making. If they wish, for example, to see the family after having seen an individual for a number of sessions, this should be carefully planned, and the therapist's goals in changing the emphasis should be explicit. A way of evaluating how far the goals of intervention have been met, and whether or not the intervention has been appropriate, should be part of the treatment. The intervention and its evaluation should happen within a planned period of time. Confused interventions by the therapist are likely to lead to a confused individual or family. In this chapter we also emphasised the responsibility of the therapist for modifying his use of psychological therapy to take account of the special needs of the elderly person. Table 8.6 summarises the factors which should be considered. The psychological approach adopted needs to be co-ordinated with appropriate medical and social interventions. It is not a panacea, but if it is neglected, many patients who could have been helped a great deal will continue to function well below their best.

Table 8.6: Factors Enhancing Therapeutic Contact with Elderly People

1. Less abstract, interpretive approach.
2. Compensate for reduction in memory for meaning.
3. Flexible session length (client comfort)
4. Flexibility of session location (client's home versus office)
5. Time-limited contract
6. Explicit, concrete, realistic goals
7. Awareness of real social and physical limitations
8. Provision of formal social resources and support
9. Interpersonal context of problem ('family' or 'institutional')
10. Active rather than passive therapist
11. Awareness of age contrast in goal setting and empathy
12. Absence of ageism in therapist.
13. Awareness of drug effects in the elderly
14. Assessment of physical factors which may exacerbate 'psychological' problems

Notes

1. Goldstein, A.P., 'Relationship - Enhancement Methods', in F.H. Kanfer and Goldstein, A.P. (eds), *Helping People Change* (Pergamon Press, Oxford, 1980).

2. Sparacino, J., 'Individual Psychotherapy with the Aged: A Selective Review', *International Review of Ageing and Human Development*, 9, 1978–79, 3, 197–220.

3. Labouvie-Vief, G. and Blanchard-Fields, F., 'Cognitive Ageing and Psychological Growth', *Ageing and Society*, 2, 1982, 2, 183–209.

4. Walker, S., 'An Investigation of the Communication of Elderly Subjects', (M Phil thesis, University of Sheffield, 1982).

5. Cohen, G. and Faulkner, D., 'Memory for Discourse in Old Age', *Discourse Processes*, 4, 1981, 253–65.

6. Taub, H.A., 'Comprehension and Memory of Prose Materials by Young and Old Adults', *Experimental Ageing Research*, 5, 1979, 3–13.

7. Ley, P., 'Psychological Studies of Doctor - Patient Communication' in S. Rachman (ed.) *Contributions to Medical Psychology* (Pergamon Press, Oxford, 1977).

8. Butler, R.N., 'Towards a Psychiatry of the Life Cycle: Implications of Sociopsychologic Studies of the Ageing Process for the Psychotherapeutic Situation', *Psychiatric Research Report*, 23, 1968, 233–48.

9. Ramsey, R.W., 'Behavioural Approaches to Bereavement', *Behaviour Research and Therapy*, 15, 1977, 2, 131–5.

10. Sholomskas, A.J., Chevron, E.S., Prusoff, B.A. and Berry, C., 'Short Term Interpersonal Theapy (IPT) with the Depressed Elderly: Case Reports and Discussion', *American Journal of Psychotherapy*, 37, 1983, 4, 552–66.

11. Watzlawick, P., Coyne, J.C., 'Depression Following Stroke: Brief, Problem-focused Family Treatment', *Family Process*, 19, 1980, 13–18.

12. Herr, J.J. and Weakland, J.H., *Counselling Elders and Their Families. Practical Techniques for Applied Gerontology* (Springer, New York, 1979).

9 NEUROPSYCHOLOGICAL ASSESSMENT AND THE ENVIRONMENT

Working with elderly people presents a particular challenge. Not only is the range of both cognitive functioning and physical health much wider, but there is also a much greater variety of life circumstances and previous life experiences than in the young. A greater degree of flexibility and a broader range of skills are therefore required to provide the best psychological help for each patient. Although the clinical psychologist has specialised training and the number of clinical psychologists working with old people is increasing, in many areas expert psychological help will not be available. It is important, therefore, that the other caring professions are aware of what clinical psychologists can do and also how they can adopt the psychological 'approach' to the assessment and management of elderly patients. In this chapter a psychological approach to elderly people who are more handicapped than those discussed in the previous chapter will be considered. The appropriate management of elderly people with chronic psychiatric illness, whether it be depression, schizophrenia, or dementia, is particularly important because of the disproportionate amount of time and resources which have to be spent in caring for them. The potential benefit in terms of the patients' and staff's well-being, as well as the economic savings, are enormous.

A careful assessment is the basis for appropriate intervention. Measures of general intelligence and personality have largely been discarded because they do not predict response to treatment and are of little help in planning management. The development of measures of more discrete but inter-related cognitive functions has proved of more practical value in work with elderly people, who have a greater prevalence of organic brain dysfunction. A neuropsychological assessment can provide a detailed picture of a person's cognitive functions — both her assets and her deficits.

Aims of the Neuropsychological Assessment

Planning Management and Treatment Programmes

Behaviour is a consequence of interactions between the individual and the environment (Figure 9.1). Where particular neuropsychological

Figure 9.1: An Interactive View of Behaviour

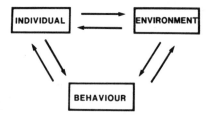

deficits exist, since it is not usually possible to remedy the organic damage by medical means, the best opportunity for management lies in changing the environment (both physical design and the way people respond to and interact with the person), in order to reduce the individual's level of handicap. The analogy of a deaf person can be used: if the physical environment is changed by providing a hearing aid, and persuading other people to talk more loudly and clearly, the level of handicap can be considerably reduced.

Neuropsychological assessment also highlights the limitations of psychiatric diagnosis. Thus, even where two individuals have the same diagnosis, for example senile dementia of the Alzheimer type (SDAT), a different pattern of deficits may be present. One, for example, may have only a mild impairment of short-term memory, but great difficulty in understanding speech, whereas another may have a severe impairment of short-term memory, but a relatively preserved ability to understand what is being said. In the former patient, the correct approach would be to provide information, guidance and help, using short sentences containing single ideas. In the latter, the patient would probably benefit more from being regularly orientated to time, person and place in a relaxed and non-threatening manner.

It is important to consider the information gained from a neuropsychological assessment in the context of the patient's general level of functioning and behaviour, both at home and on the ward. Rating scales, such as the Behaviour Rating Scale (BRS) of Clifton Assessment Procedures for the Elderly (CAPE), provide a quick and easy measure of an elderly person's general level of functioning and behaviour.[1] The BRS consists of 18 individual items divided into four subscales: physical disability, apathy, communication difficulties and social disturbance. It is not uncommon to find a relative absence of neuropsychological dysfunction, yet a poor score on the BRS, indicating a high level of dependence. This suggests that an elderly person is not functioning at the level she should or could be and the reasons for this can be explored and possibly rectified.

It should be noted that no standard rating scale of behaviour can be regarded as ideal. One problem, which arises from making such scales brief enough to be used routinely and efficiently, is that subscale items become insensitive in measuring change. For example, the incontinence item on the BRS is scored nil points for never incontinent, one point for incontinent once or twice a week and two points for incontinent three or more times a week. Thus a clinically significant improvement, a patient who was incontinent eight times a day becoming incontinent only once a day, would not be 'measured'.

Diagnosis

An elderly person's mental state is the result of a complex interaction of medical, psychological and social factors. For example, elderly people may present as confused if they are depressed, medically ill, suffering from sensory deprivation, or dementing. In these circumstances it is not always easy to decide which is the appropriate psychiatric diagnosis. A neuropsychological assessment can indicate whether or not there is an organic brain lesion, helping to distinguish a depressive illness from dementia. It can also suggest whether this is part of a global deterioration, as in dementia, or whether it is a relatively discrete deficit indicative of a tumour or cerebral infarction.

The Neuropsychological Assessment

It is important, when making a neuropsychological assessment, to take account of the patient's educational level, as a well-educated person with a functional deficit may still perform better than an uneducated person on tests of that function. There are other important considerations when assessing elderly people. Normal elderly people perform considerably worse than younger people on certain tests of cognitive function. The reasons for this are varied and range from actual impairment of ability to failure to see the significance of the tests and therefore failure to make an effort.

The detection of various deficits is often a matter of fine clinical judgement, not only because of age-related changes in cognitive function, but also because of the relative lack of studies looking at cognitive function in normal elderly people. One exception to this is a study which looked at drawing disability as a measure of constructional apraxia in elderly people with dementia.[2] As well as providing valuable data about the qualitative and quantitative differences in simple spontaneous drawings and copies made by elderly people with and without dementia, it was found that the drawing of a cube was not a useful discriminative test, as normal elderly test subjects also performed poorly.[3]

Qualitative Versus Quantitative

In practice, clinical psychologists have been split between the quantitative and qualitative approach to the neuropsychological assessment of the elderly person. When it is considered that one well-known neuropsychological test battery takes some five hours to administer, the problems of the quantitative approach become apparent. As one eminent psychologist wrote many such tests are only useful for 'battering the individual'. The advantages of the qualitative approach are:

1) That formal assessments over extended periods, which are likely to be poorly tolerated and stressful experiences for the more elderly and infirm, can be avoided. Taking the patient's personal history in a sympathetic way can reveal a good deal about memory and cognitive functioning. An ordinary magazine can be used as an unthreatening way of testing reading, object and colour recognition, and the use of appropriate words to describe objects.[4]

2) It is frequently impossible to use formal, quantitative measures when the patient's neuropsychological and psychiatric state is most in doubt. Faced with a chair-fast woman who replies to nearly every question with the answer 'don't know', even the use of a simple assessment measure, the CAPE orientation and information (O/I) scale, is impossible. In one such case, the fact that the woman concerned remembered the psychologist's name at the next meeting two days later provided some useful evidence about her ability to learn new information. When formal tests are impossible the patient should be observed in everyday activities, hypotheses made about what specific deficits appear to be present, and then specific informal 'tests' should be devised to confirm or deny their presence. It might be noted that this is not routinely done in acute ward settings. One of the authors was referred a woman who appeared inconsistently orientated, with circumscribed but coherent speech, who refused to be formally interviewed. It was clear from brief observation and interaction with her that she was grossly receptively impaired, having little understanding of speech and covering this up with a well-

developed repertoire of stock phrases and responsiveness to social cues. During her two months on the ward no member of that team had noted the possibility of the presence of a receptive dysphasia.

3) Some areas of neuropsychological function are particularly difficult to measure with quantitative assessment procedures. This problem is further compounded when the qualitative features of the dysfunction are similar to other psychiatric disorders. The function of the frontal lobes is a case in point. Dysfunction in this area of the brain may result in a wide range of different behavioural consequences, many of these difficult to quantify. It is not uncommon to find emotional lability misconstrued as indicating a clinical depression, whilst the presence of disinhibition can lead to a misdiagnosis of hypomania or schizophrenia (and vice versa). Luria who pioneered research into frontal lobe function has suggested a range of qualitative assessment procedures which might be used to detect frontal dysfunction.[5]

In emphasising the importance of a qualitative assessment in the elderly, the importance of quantitative assessment must not be ignored. (For example, the use of the CAPE BRS to relate and adjust staffing levels according to the level of dependancy found in each Social Service residential home, would allow a major rationalisation of the present residential provision for elderly people.) In most cases a good clinician will use a combined approach. Unfortunately, it has been the author's experience that when well-standardised and predictive non-threatening tests of specific abilities are available, e.g. CAPE or Hodkinson scales for orientation, clinicians often use idiosyncratic tests of dubious validity, yet fail to recognise important qualitative features of the patient's behaviour, which would help to clarify diagnosis. One answer lies in improving the basic level of knowledge of all professions about neuropsychological dysfunction and its implications for management.

Brief definitions of some of the principal neuropsychological deficits are given in Table 9.1. Appropriate education and intellectual levels, reasonable sensory and motor function and familiarity of the test objects is assumed. Much more detailed accounts of neuropsychological assessment[6,7] and some implications for management[8,9] are available to interested readers. The following case-histories illustrate some of the implications these various neuropsychological deficits have for management, treatment and diagnosis.

Table 9.1: Brief Definitions of the Principal Neuropsychological Deficits

Aphasia/Dysphasia
This refers to a difficulty in the use of language
Nominal aphasia — the person is able to recognise an object but has difficulty naming it appropriately
Receptive dysphasia — a person may have relatively normal speech but has difficulty in understanding what is being said to her
Expressive — this is an impairment in the production of speech which can range from complete loss to shortened sentences and mild word-finding problems

Agnosia
This refers to an impairment in the ability to recognise things
Visual agnosia — a person is not only unable to name an object but will not be able to recognise it for what it is (unless she uses another sense, e.g. touch)
Spatial agnosia — a person is unable to find her way round familiar surroundings. There may also be distortion in the memory of spatial relationships of her surroundings

Apraxia
This is the impairment of the ability to carry out voluntary and purposeful movements (excluding other causes such as muscle weakness and failure of comprehension)
Constructional apraxia — in this case there is a difficulty in putting together parts to make a whole, e.g. when making a simple drawing
Dressing apraxia — there is a particular difficulty in dressing, e.g. in fastening buttons or tying shoe laces

Frontal
Deficits in this area result in a variety of qualitative signs such as perseveration and emotional lability

Memory
One simple distinction made is between short-term memory (memory for recent events) and long-term memory. An impairment in short-term memory is identified by assessing a person's ability to learn and recall new material over short-time intervals

Acquired Knowledge
Difficulties with reading (dyslexia), writing (dysgraphia) and arithmetic (acalculia), which are all acquired abilities, can arise from particular cerebral lesions

Subcortical
This is characterised by forgetfulness, slowness of thought, personality change and the impaired ability to manipulate acquired knowledge

Case 9.1:

Mr G.B. was aged 77 and lived at home with his wife. He was admitted to a medical ward suffering from a suspected occipital stroke. We were consulted about the advisability of discharging him home to his wife after he had episodes of kicking and punching the nursing staff while on the ward. He returned home on our advice, but unfortunately Valium, prescribed by his GP to help his sleep disturbance, made him confused and bedridden. He was admitted to our acute psychiatric ward, returned home after a three-week detailed assessment, and attends our day hospital once a week so that his wife has a break from caring. The management plan shown in Table 9.2 considerably reduced problem behaviours both on the ward and at the day hospital. Although he initially improved over the months he has shown an intermittent decline, probably indicative of a multi-infarct dementia, and Mr G.B. and his wife are likely to need long-term and increasing support if they are to manage at home. The nurses in day hospital now know Mr G.B. well and have come to appreciate that one of his retained functions is a sharp sense of humour.

Table 9.2: Mr G.B.'s Management Plan

Neuropsychological	Management implications
Right visual field defect	Staff should approach from the left at all times, whether for conversation or to request something
Poor short-term memory	Routinely provide reality-orientated information and cues, e.g. 'My name is Sheila, it is 12 o'clock and lunch is being served. Can I show you the way?'
Visual agnosia and astereognosis (tactile)	He will find activities depending on vision and tactile cues difficult and frustrating. Concentrate on other activities such as music
Inappropriate behaviours	Reinforce acceptable behaviour with staff time and interest, and reduce reinforcement when he behaves appropriately
ALSO	
Mr G.B. has insight (but approach also applies if little or no insight)	Treat as an adult; allow choice. Listen and respond appropriately to his requests. Be empathetic about his loss of abilities
Preserved social skills	Appropriate use of his dry sense of humour

Case History 9.2:

Mr D.N. was a 66-year-old man living at home, supported by relatives who lived next door. He was admitted for assessment following increasing self-neglect. His relatives supported 'slowness rather than silliness'. He had been an epileptic since the age of 18. A comparison of the degree and extent of these deficits (Table 9.3) with his score on the Modified Crichton Rating Scale (similar to the BRS) indicated that his behaviour and general functioning were better than might be expected. However, it was still thought that he would not be able to cope with living alone. With his agreement, he was eventually discharged to an old people's home.

One important aspect of Mr D.N.'s management was for the staff to be aware of his slowness in carrying out tasks due to subcortical involvement. If this slowness had been interpreted as an inability to carry out or complete the task, the staff might have intervened inappropriately and effectively 'untrained' his self-care skills, making him highly dependent and institutionalised. Because staff at the old people's home were fully informed as to the nature and extent of his deficits, they were able to implement a level of care appropriate to his needs.

Table 9.3: The Degree and Extent of Mr D.N.'s Deficits

Neuropsychological deficits	Management implications
Nominal aphasia	Staff to use cueing, e.g. to say first letter or syllable of word he cannot find
Receptive dysphasia	Requests, commands and conversations to include only short simple sentences with one idea at a time
Subcortical involvement (slowness, occasional irritable outbursts)	Allow him time to complete tasks

Case 9.3:

Mrs E.S. a 67-year-old woman, was brought to the hospital by her husband, who reported marked changes in her behaviour and personality in recent months. She muttered obscenities to herself, made unusual sexual advances towards her husband and had night-time singing sessions. A psychiatric diagnosis could not easily be made. Table 9.4 shows the results of a neuropsychological investigation. The findings of isolated frontal signs in the absence of any global impairment of intellect or other clear-cut deficits indicated an isolated lesion in the frontal lobes. Further investigations included a CAT scan. This was within normal limits, but did indicate a possible small shadow in the frontal region. Her mental state was closely monitored by our community nurse and a CAT scan was repeated after three months. It was concluded from this that the shadow in the frontal region

Table 9.4: Results of Mrs E.S.'s Neuropsychological
Investigation

Neuropsychological findings	Implications
Premorbid IQ ≡ present IQ	No global intellectual deterioration
Frontal signs	Frontal lobe lesion
i) Failure on motor sequencing	
ii) Slight perseveration	
iii) Emotional lability	
iv) Lack of insight	
Possible nominal aphasia	Result not clear-cut

represented a congenital abnormality, the behavioural effects of which had been unmasked by ageing. The use of night-time medication and the support and advice of the community nurse led to an improvement in Mrs E.S.'s general behaviour allowing her and her husband to socialise more, but her long-term management remains difficult.

Detailed assessment of neuropsychological functioning and appropriate management measures can often be a way of producing marked improvements in the behaviour and quality of life of individuals who might otherwise be written off as unhelpable.

Contingency Management

As well as considering the implications of possible neuropsychological deficits for the environment, situational factors of another kind should be considered. These factors have been called 'contingencies', and contingency management has made a unique contribution to the well-being of mentally handicapped people who have been shown to have the ability to learn a wide range of skills, given the appropriate situational factors. More disturbed elderly people, including those with organic brain pathology, may benefit from the use of an appropriate contingency management programme.

There are complicated ethical issues involved in the use of contingency management as the people most likely to be treated by this method are often unable to speak for their own needs. Anyone using contingency management procedures should therefore be sure that the elderly person's well-being is the primary consideration. Detailed accounts of the applications and ethical problems of contingency management with more handicapped people are available.[10,11]

Special Considerations

Older people, like children, tend to be more dependent on other people, often close relatives. This sometimes leads to them being *inappropriately* treated like children. Helpers may perceive an old person as being deliberately awkward, when in fact her behaviour is conditioned by a mental illness, or maladaptive learned behaviour. In contingency management the attitude of helpers is all-important, as their reactions may unwittingly be encouraging the behaviours about which they complain.

In an old person a particular 'problem behaviour' may have many different causes, only some of which may be amenable to the contingency management approach. This is illustrated in Table 9.5 for the problem of urinary incontinence.

Table 9.5: Problem Behaviour — Urinary Incontinence in an Elderly Mildly Confused Person

Reason	Solution
1　Medical (e.g. Urinary Tract Infection)	Treat medical condition
2　*Incontinence being reinforced by staff*	*Rewarding periods of dryness*
3　*Cannot find toilet (short-term memory impairment)*	*Practice, use of a variety of cues, and signposting*
4　Cannot recognise toilet (visual agnosia)	Use a colour code, e.g. only red in unit is toilet doors
5　Cannot get to toilet in time (mobility)	Increase availability of toilet
6　Stress incontinence	Pelvic floor muscle exercises
7　*Cannot dress or undress*	*Practise dressing/undressing skills*
8　Toilet uncomfortable (e.g. commode seat-top missing)	Make more comfortable
9　*Lack of motivation. Severe depression*	*Encourage and reinforce successful toileting and dryness*
10　Cannot understand verbal instructions to toilet (receptive aphasia)	Use alternative cue, e.g. visual
11　Cannot express need for toilet (expressive aphasia)	Staff sensitive to individual's attempt to communicate needs. Knowledge of individual's routine

Italics indicate that a contingency management approach should be used.

This example also shows the complex nature of elderly people's problems. Sadly it is still the rule rather than the exception to find pejorative labels such as 'attention-seeking', 'aggressive' or 'manipulative' used to describe elderly people in medical or residential care notes. These labels do little more than denigrate elderly people and may lead to them being treated in ways which provoke more distressed behaviour. Pragmatically, such labels provide little or no information which can be used to help change behaviour. The authors have heard the label 'confused' used to describe someone who cannot find the way around a ward or to the toilet, who does not accept she is in hospital, who tries to 'escape' regularly to see her husband (who has been dead five years). Clearly, only a more detailed description of the problem behaviour and circumstances surrounding it can allow the development of a constructive management plan.

The Concept of Reinforcement

A particular behaviour is more likely to recur if it is positively reinforced or rewarded. What at first sight appears to be a negative reinforcement or 'punishment' may in fact turn out to be a positive reinforcement. This is illustrated in Figure 9.2 which shows how an elderly confused person might develop behaviour problems. As the person becomes more confused, helpers find it less easy to converse with her and spend more time elsewhere. One study showed nurses interacted with more orientated individuals 15 per cent of the time, but only an average of 5.6 per cent of the time with more disorientated individuals.[12] This reduction in input leads to an increase in the elderly person's confusion and eventually she may, for example, strip off in public as a result of her confusion. This immediately results in a great deal of attention from helpers, involving dressing and, often, reprimands. In the context of lack of attention at other times, this reaction to the patient's inappropriate behaviour is positively reinforcing, and hence the behaviour is more likely to recur.

On the other hand, when an elderly confused person behaves appropriately, for example using dinner utensils rather than fingers to eat a meal, or sitting quietly in the corner of the room, or urinating appropriately in the toilet, there is often an immediate withdrawal of attention. Thus appropriate behaviour results in helpers leaving immediately and getting on with other work while inappropriate behaviour tends to be followed by increased attention.

In institutional settings, with a shortage of staff and a lack of structured activities throughout the day, the essentially well-meaning action

Figure 9.2: Model of the Development of a Problem Behaviour in Confused Elderly People

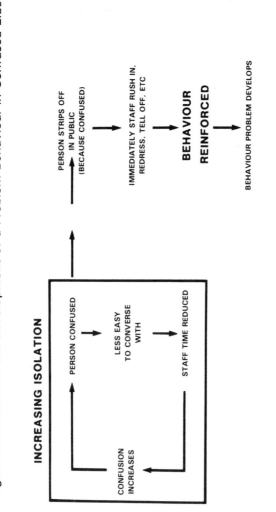

Figure 9.3: The Steps in Contingency Management

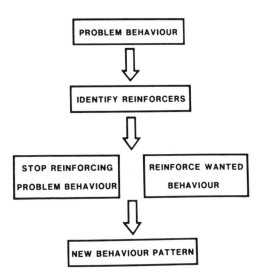

of staff can thus be the basis for an elderly confused person developing a wide range of behaviour problems to the point of becoming 'unmanageable'. In planning contingency management to undo this kind of problem behaviour, a logical series of steps can be followed (Figure 9.3). The target behaviour is first identified and then those factors in the environment which are reinforcing this behaviour are also identified, usually by direct, unobtrusive observation of the elderly person in the environment where the problem behaviour occurs. The next stage involves stopping the reinforcement of the problem behaviour, while at the same time starting to reinforce wanted behaviour, so that eventually a new pattern of behaviour emerges. The following case-studies illustrate this approach.

Case 9.4:

Mrs M.L. was an 87-year-old single lady who returned to an old people's home after recovering from a broken femur. She had a diagnosis of moderate dementia, probably SDAT, was rather deaf and suffered from cataracts. She was referred because of increasing confusion and various problem behaviours, which included faecal soiling and smearing, using her fingers for eating and not attempting to co-operate with walking practice or the use of a Zimmer frame.

Whilst a detailed interview with the staff clearly indicated what factors might be involved in these problem behaviours, it was decided

Table 9.6: Behavioural Observation of Mrs M.L. during One Meal-time Period

Observations	Programme
1 Staff only interact to do things to her or in response to unpleasant behaviour	Regular periods of ten minutes during day to be spent dealing with her in a pleasant manner. Only following periods of quiet or adaptive behaviour
2 Confused	Re-orientate her to time, person and place regularly during 1
3 Staff do not approach her in a manner to take account of her poor hearing and eyesight	Demonstrate use of touch, close visual face-to-face contact to staff
4 Staff do not respond to her verbal requests	Increase staff awareness of her verbal requests
5 Little staff time and praise given when she performs appropriately	Increase positive reinforcement of succcessful behaviour
6 Staff time and attention raised when she behaves appropriately	Decrease staff and resident attention following inappropriate behaviour

to observe Mrs M.L. directly in certain situations, for example over lunch. Table 9.6 provides a list of the observations made in one meal-time period.

This information, together with the staff's comments, provided the basis for planning a treatment programme to reduce Mrs M.L.'s problem behaviours, and to increase her level of independence and appropriate behaviour. The treatment programme involved both contingency management and the use of reality orientation. In practice, detailed instructions are given to staff in any particular problem situation.

Over the first two weeks of the programme Mrs M.L.'s problem behaviours gradually reduced. However, at this point she was admitted to hospital for an operation on her cataracts and the programme was discontinued until she was discharged. When the programme was reinstituted, the improvement continued, probably helped by her improved vision.

An additional effect of the programme was her improved interaction with other residents. Some of the residents had presumably noticed one of the authors and other staff members responding to Mrs M.L. in an appropriate reality-orientated manner, reminding her of where she was, what time of day it was, etc., and they began to do the same. Thus, Mrs M.L. also gained input from other residents during the day which helped to reduce her level of confusion. She maintained this progress over a six-month period until her sudden death.

Case 9.5:

Mrs B.U. was a 75-year-old widow with a 20-year history of depression. Prior to her most recent admission she had been progressing well, attending the day hospital on a regular basis. There she appeared to benefit both from group cognitive therapy and from the development of various skills, such as cooking. However, her son, who provided considerable care and support in the community and lived nearby, continued to be extremely concerned about the demands his mother placed on him. This had reached the point where his marriage had began to suffer.

Following a brief admission it was decided that the clinical psychologist would work closely with Mrs B.U.'s son to try to see if her improved ability to cope in the day hospital setting could be made to generalise to her situation at home. Both direct observations of Mrs B.U. on the ward and a detailed interview with the son provided sufficient information on which to base a programme. On the evening of her discharge the psychologist visited her at home to find both Mrs B.U. and her son near to tears and her son asking for her to be readmitted.

Table 9.7 shows some of the findings from observation and interview. Perhaps the most significant finding was the way in which Mrs B.U., by the things she said, would draw people into destructive interactions with her. Thus even if she could undertake a task successfully she would either ask for help or say that she did not know what to do and when people performed these tasks for her, she both lost a skill and lost further confidence in her own abilities. The programme involved redistributing the amount of time the son was spending to reinforce positive aspects of her behaviour and reducing his time and input when, for example, she was shouting for him. This helped him cope with his own emotions and in turn produced a positive effect on his relationship with his mother.

A further aspect of the programme which the son himself developed was to set small but increasing goals towards independence. Thus over the weeks she progressed from insisting that he bathed her to bathing herself when he was there, through to his putting up a hand rail and her eventually being able to take a bath whenever she wanted. She continued to improve gradually and the level of support was reduced to the point where the son could spend time with his own family in a constructive way and was not emotionally drained when he returned

Table 9.7: Findings from Observing and Interviewing Mrs B.U.

Observations	Programme
1 Constantly asking for help (unnecessarily) and saying: 'What do I do?'	Son not to do everything for her and to respond verbally by indicating he thinks she can succeed
2 Problem behaviours such as shouting	Reduce time and reinforcement immediately following these incidents
3 Low level of self-help skills at home	Set gradually increasing goals and reinforce any successes with extra time and input
4 Loneliness	Encourage her involvement in a variety of social situations — apply for sheltered accommodation
5 Better performance at day hospital than at home	Close liaison with day hospital to have reliable information about her potential capabilities at home

home. In the next year Mrs B.U., completely of her own volition, applied for a sheltered flatlet, as she had never been happy with the house she was living in. As this was near her son's house and she was making a decision for herself it was decided to fully support her application. However, when the move did come it proved disastrous when, because of the strain of having to cope with a new situation, her old problem behaviours re-emerged. Unfortunately, her good neighbours reinforced her inappropriate behaviour and encouraged her helplessness through their caring efforts. The situation was resolved when she was found a place in an old people's home. There she made friends with another elderly resident and became her constant companion, even sharing the bedroom with her. Her problem behaviours gradually diminished and she continues to lead a much happier existence.

Thus, contingency management can help in both the institutional setting and at home, in helping relatives to cope with old people with problem behaviours. Unfortunately, in institutional settings, and especially in old people's homes, the lack of special staff training means that inappropriate behaviours often continue to be reinforced. The approach of contingency management can often improve the quality of life, both for the old person and their helpers. It deserves to be more widely used.

Physical Environment

So far the importance of the environment as represented by the carer, whether relative, support worker or therapist, has been emphasised. The physical design of environments is equally important in influencing the elderly person's functional ability. The effect of ageing is to reduce the body's spare capacity for coping with change, thus while a young person may have 95 per cent capacity in reserve, an older person may have only 5 per cent or less spare. Carrying out a task which calls on 10 per cent of this spare capacity will go unnoticed by the younger person, but will cause the elderly person severe distress. The net effect of this reduction in capacity is to make the elderly person increasingly dependent on the environment. It is a sad reflection on our society that we design environments for our elderly people which not only deny them the basic comforts and rights we take for granted ourselves but that also take little account of this increased dependence. The physical environments we expect our elderly people to live in are little short of scandalous. Before readers decide this is an over-reaction they should consider a study which looked at seating for residents in three Social Services homes for the elderly.[13] In this residents who were chair-fast with the seating provided (n = 39) were identified. It was found that 77 per cent of these elderly people could rise unaided when provided with a DHSS recommended chair. Nearly £2,000 had been spent on unsuitable chairs in these residential homes, and had current guidelines been used in the selection of chairs, staff would have been saved a minimum of 300 lifts a day for meals and toileting. There is no reason to suppose that this finding would not be repeated throughout the country. The authors acknowledge that designing environments is not easy. Returning to the previous example, producing an adequately designed chair would involve the consideration of a minimum of 21 factors and even then, no one chair would be suitable for all elderly people. It is impossible in the space available to provide a comprehensive account of this subject, rather our aim is to sensitise readers to the range and complexity of factors involved and to stimulate ideas about how they might improve the environments they work in with elderly people.

Sensory Deficits

Ageing leads to increasing loss of function in the various senses. With regard to the physical environment the most important of these are visual, auditory and, though not strictly a sense, motor ability. A few examples of the implications of changes in visual function illustrate the variety of different environmental factors.

Colour Fading. With increasing lens opaqueness colours tend to fade, some colours such as blue and green fading more. Typically institutional settings have soft pastel colours for their decor, which the elderly person is likely to see as grey. How many of our readers would choose to live in a totally grey environment? Indeed when it is considered that integrity of brain function depends on an adequate level of stimulation and that the effects of ageing will have reduced input from other senses, the importance of selecting colours which are three or four shades brighter can be understood. Within residential homes or sheltered flatlets, this problem can be ameliorated by allowing elderly people to select their own decorations.

Lighting Levels. An improved light level will facilitate the performance of various activities amongst the young and old. However, elderly people benefit significantly more.[14] Whilst architects often get lighting levels right, an example of one common design fault is that of transition lighting. Thus because the elderly eye adjusts less quickly to changes in light levels, moving from a room which is artificially lit to an area which is even well lit by natural lighting can be rather like the experience you or I would have when walking into an unlit cellar. When the area being entered is a stairway, this becomes more than just stressful for the elderly person, it becomes a life-threatening hazard. Too often it has been the authors' experience when visiting private residential homes, for example, that stairway lighting is either inadequate, or off, to save money. Rather than relying on chance, one solution to prevent lighting at transition points being routinely switched off (by residents or staff) would be to make the on/off switch particularly inaccessible.

Visual Disturbance. Perceptual effects not normally experienced by younger people may be experienced by elderly people because of the interactive effects of sensory and motor deficit. Some elderly people tend to stoop when walking and thus, rather than looking forward, look down to the floor. Walking looking down at geometric or intricate floral patterns (as is found on some flotex) can produce perceptual disturbances, such as the floor appearing to move, particularly if the surface is uneven. This may in turn lead to somatic feelings such as queasiness and reduce the already shaky confidence of someone who is unsteady on her feet. Such patterns should be avoided in corridor flooring, but may be used in small room areas where walking is limited. The reader may like to experience this effect for themselves by selecting a corridor with geometric pattern floor and walking along, looking down.

Rather than considering any further examples of the effects of sensory and motor deficit, the implications for environmental design for elderly people who suffer from dementia will be examined next.

Cognitive Deficits

Earlier in this chapter the range and variety of neuropsychological deficits present in dementia were considered and some examples of how changes in staff behaviour reduced the effects of these cognitive handicaps were given. (See Tables 9.2 and 9.3.) The design of the physical environment is also important in either reducing or magnifying the effects of such handicaps.

Short-term Memory. Difficulties in being able to learn or retain new information can profoundly affect our ability to cope with everyday life. The interactive effect of short-term memory with the environment can be simply illustrated. Consider for a moment how you can find the date on an ordinary calendar which displays every day of a particular month? Quite simply you can work out what day it is only by knowing roughly what day it is. Someone with a short-term memory problem often does not know roughly when it is and this environmental aid becomes useless.

Even for those with milder levels of handicap, a central problem in providing a 'prosthetic' or artifical memory aid is that of being able to remember to use or even find the aid. This can be overcome when regular support is available, for example, by the use of a white board fixed in the person's living room or kitchen. The elderly person can be taught to go to this board when uncertain about something, and its successful use depends on it being changed daily to provide orientating information such as date, and also important tasks or events of that day. The authors know of one lady who during the start of an early dementia began to label important items in her home and developed a rigid routine which, for example, involved crossing off each day on her monthly calendar. Recent research in providing community support for those with dementia has indicated that the success of such support depends on encouraging and facilitating a very set routine geared towards the individual's particular needs.[15] Whenever these routines are disrupted by, for example, bad weather, they become difficult to reinstate and the outcome is often hospital admission. Such findings reinforce the importance of the early detection and support of those with dementia.

Institutional settings are notoriously poor at providing orientating information to reduce the effects of short-term memory difficulties. Important areas such as the residents' sleeping bay, the dining room, sitting room and toilets should all be clearly labelled. Where possible alternative cues should be used, thus a toilet door should not only be labelled 'Ladies' and 'Gents', but should have simple representative pictures posted on them and be colour coded, for example, bright red. Thus someone who cannot read, for example, may still have an understandable cue from which to learn where the toilet is. Simplicity and ease of understanding should be the key notes of all such design features. For example, an orientating aid such as a clock may be rendered useless, for a confused person, by the use of Roman numerals. It must be remembered that the presence of such cues is not sufficient, but that the patient or resident must be encouraged to use the cues on every possible occasion. Furthermore, one study has shown that having sessions involving active practice at finding key areas on a ward improved some elderly people's ability to find their way around, regardless of the severity of dementia.[16] How can people with learning difficulties be expected to learn their way to the toilet when they are always taken to it? It is much harder to find your way back to somewhere, when you have only been taken there as a passive 'passenger', even without a short-term memory problem.

Interaction

The design of physical environments not only has effects on the individual but may also influence the behaviour of groups of elderly people living together. This can be illustrated in relation to interaction between elderly people. It is all too common to see a group of elderly people on a ward, or in a residential home, sat around the edges of a large open-plan room, see Figure 9.4. Typically there is almost no interaction between these elderly people. This is not surprising when it is likely many have reduced hearing and poor mobility. Reduced hearing makes conversation particularly difficult when sat side by side to someone and poor mobility makes the strategy of turning side on, or even moving to a better position, unlikely. A further common feature in such settings, the booming television, reduces the possibility of interaction still further. Attempts to improve the situation by putting chairs around tables (Figure 9.5) generally fail, as the chairs 'magically' resume their positions around the wall overnight (Figure 9.4). Figure 9.6 shows that relatively inexpensive physical changes can prevent this problem. Thus, dividing off an area of room and blocking off wall areas by the use of furniture, plants, etc. not only make it physically impossible to put chairs in positions which

Figure 9.4: Interaction and Physical Design: Typical Open-plan Day Area leading to Reduced Interaction

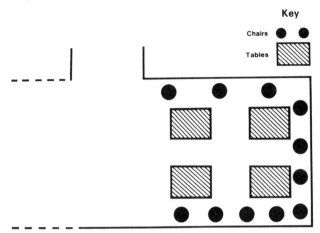

Figure 9.5: Interaction and Physical Design: Change in Physical Position of Chairs can improve Interaction but Rarely Lasts

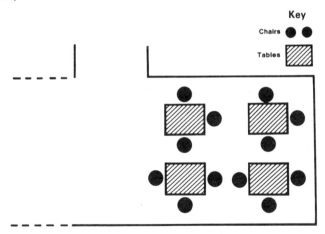

reduce the potential for interaction, but also foster a homely environment. Clearly interaction with other people or materials, is also dependent on, for example, choice of activity, access to other elderly people of similar 'ability', reinforcement, encouragement and reminders by staff, but unless the permanent physical environment is designed to promote interaction even the most enthusiastic of staff efforts will be likely to

Figure 9.6: Interaction and Physical Design: Changes which improve Interaction can be made Permanent, are Relatively Inexpensive and allow Personalisation of the Environment

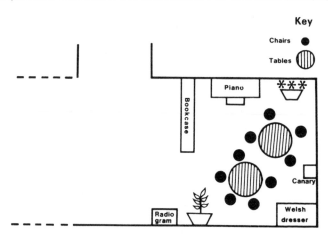

fail. One practical example of the effect of simple environmental changes on interaction is given by Davies and Snaith.[17] This example illustrates a further important concept to be considered when designing environments, that every design feature has a dual quality, i.e. that of having both good and bad consequences. Thus designing a room to promote interaction also reduces the opportunity for being by oneself, a need we all have on occasion. Such needs can be catered for by the provision of a small quiet room away from the main sitting area. The authors believe that every effort should be made to maximise the elderly person's choice in this manner. However, since the sensory and motor deficits of ageing do tend to prevent interaction, it does make sense that the elderly person has to make an active choice not to interact (by going to a quiet area), rather than being placed in a situation where interaction is difficult whatever they do.

Dignity and Self-esteem

It is possible to control more subtle psychological aspects of the environment such as privacy through the manipulation of physical design. Many people reading this will have seen elderly people, on hospital wards, being toileted in public view, because the toilet doors have not been closed adequately. Rather than blaming nursing staff, who are often overworked and underpaid, the responsibility is more properly placed with the architects who designed the wards. If the toilet is designed as in Figure

Figure 9.7: Toilet Design: Increased Probability of Public Toileting

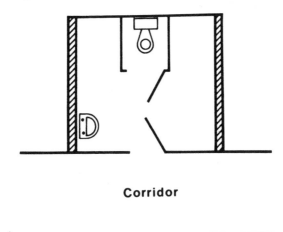

Corridor

Figure 9.8: Decreased Probability of Public Toileting

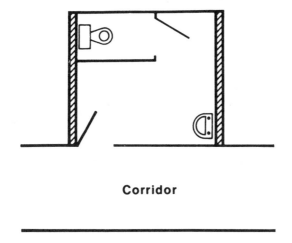

Corridor

9.7 it can be guaranteed that patients' privacy for toileting will be reduced at some time or other. However, if toilet areas are designed as in Figure 9.8 the patients' privacy when being toileted is almost certain to be maintained. Elderly people are routinely subjected to experiences, such as public toileting, few of us would willingly accept. The cumulative effects on the elderly person's dignity and self-esteem can only be guessed at.

Care Staff Needs

The well-being of elderly people in an institutional setting depends upon their interactions with the care staff. If the physical environment is not designed to support the needs of these staff, then the ease with which they can carry out important duties regarding the patients' care will be affected. Returning to the first example given in this section regarding chair design, the physical demands of 300 extra lifts/day must influence the staff's ability or willingness to meet the psychological needs of the residents. It certainly leaves less time available for other aspects of care. One important duty for nurses is to maintain discreet, but careful, observation of patients on their ward. The authors know of hospital wards designed within the last ten years which, by having numerous side rooms off a long corridor, prevent nursing staff from giving adequate levels of observation. One can speculate on the effects such poor designs have, for example on accidental fall rates amongst elderly inpatients. Figure 9.9 shows part of a day hospital in which the careful positioning of the staff base allowed the supervision of two of the three patient areas through windows A and B, and allowed the observation of patients or others entering and leaving the day hospital through door C. This was a refurbished building rather than being purpose built and shows that even when the possibilities are limited a satisfactory solution can be achieved.

An important factor which should be considered by those involved in developing or planning new physical resources for the elderly is that of size. The larger the facility in terms of numbers of patients it caters for, the harder it is to design a satisfactory physical environment. There are also increasing organisational problems. It is much harder to achieve individual care and management for a group of 30 elderly people than for a group of 15. Elderly people with widely differing problems and abilities should not have to be routinely placed together, as happens at present, because facilities are too large. It seems likely that a humane solution to the care of some groups of elderly people, for example those with dementia involving significant frontal pathology will depend on the provision of very small residential homes. Some of the behaviour which arises from their frontal pathology, for example sexual disinhibition, makes it impossible to care for them in larger settings, because of the distress it causes to other residents and relatives.

Throughout this book, the importance of the style and content of communication between the 'carer' and the elderly person has been stressed. What are often less well recognised and less easy to control are the communications which any particular environment, whether residential old peoples' home, day hospital or acute admission ward, makes to each

Figure 9.9: Example of Part of a Refurbished Day Hospital in which Nursing Staff are allowed Good Observation of Patient Areas and of Entrance/Exits

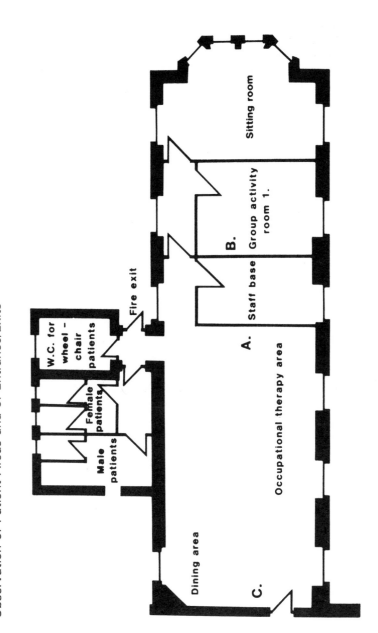

elderly person entering it. Every setting communicates (intentionally or not) information about what is expected of the elderly person in terms of, for example, independence, decision-making, control, responsibility and activity.

This information may be communicated in quite a subtle manner. Thus, in a psychogeriatric day hospital, having a regular daily meeting involving elderly attenders deciding with staff on the programme of activities is likely to promote control and independence. Planning the activity programme without involving the elderly attenders can only set up the expectation that no decisions are required of them and push them further into dependency. Some evidence exists about the effects of such variables on the well-being of elderly people.[18,19] Those caring for elderly people in such settings should look carefully at 'what' and 'how' their environments communicate to elderly people attending or living there and if necessary make changes. This aspect of the environment should no more be left to chance than each individual programme of care.

Conclusion

We have put forward the view that elderly people who suffer from chronic conditions such as dementia have the same rights of dignity and independence within their remaining capabilities as elderly people who do not suffer from these conditions. There is no one correct approach to meet all the situations we might face in working with these more handicapped groups of people and it is often hard to represent their individual needs adequately when faced with pressures from the institution or relatives. A psychological approach which centres on the importance of the environment in determining behaviour and stresses multidisciplinary involvement in both assessment and management is a firm basis from which to meet these needs.

Notes

1. Pattie, A.H. and Gilleard, C.J. *Clifton Assessment Procedures for the Elderly* (NFER-Nelson, Windsor, 1979).

2. Moore, V. and Wyke, M.A. 'Drawing Disability in Patients with Senile Dementia', *Psychological Medicine*, 14, 1984, 1, 97–105.

3. Moore, V.R. 'Analysis of Drawing Ability in Adults with Dementia' (M Phil thesis, University of London, 1981).

4. Holden, U.P. and Woods, R.T. *Reality Orientation. Psychological Approaches to the 'Confused' Elderly* (Churchill Livingstone, Edinburgh, 1982).

5. Luria, A.R., Pribram, K.H. and Homskaya, E.D. 'An Experimental Analysis of the Behavioural Disturbance Produced by a Left Frontal Arachnoidal Endothelioma (Meningioma)', *Neuropsychologia*, 2, 1964, 257–80.

6. Walsh, R.W. *Neuropsychology. A Clinical Approach* (Churchill Livingstone, Edinburgh, 1978).

7. Warrington, E.K. 'Neurological Deficits', in P. Miller (ed.), *The Psychological Assessment of Mental and Physical Handicaps* (Tavistock Publications associated with Methuen, London, 1976).

8. Church, M.A. 'Forgotten Something', *Nursing Times*, 24–30 July 1985, 23–4.

9. Church, M.A. 'Cues to Clarity', *Nursing Times*, 31 July–6 August 1985, 35–7.

10. Rimm, D.C. and Masters, J.C. *Behaviour Therapy — Techniques and Empirical Findings* (Academic Press, London, 1974).

11. Barker, P.J. *Behaviour Therapy Nursing* (Croom Helm, London, 1982).

12. Browne, K. 'Confusion in the Elderly', *Nursing*, 2, 1984, 24, 698–705.

13. Finlay, O.E., Bayles, T.B., Rosen, C. and Milling, J. 'Effects of Chair Design, Age and Cognitive Status on Mobility', *Age and Ageing*, 12, 1983, 4, 329–31.

14. Guth, S.K., Eastmann, A.A. and McNellis, J.F. 'Lighting Requirements for Older Workers', *Illumination Engineering*, 11, 1956, 656–60.

15. Challis, D. and Davies, B. 'Community Care: A Development in the Home Care for the Elderly' in J. Grimley Evans and F.I. Caird, *Advanced Geriatric Medicine* (Pitman, London, 1984).

16. Hanley, I.G. 'The Use of Sign Posts and Active Training to Modify Ward Disorientation in Elderly Patients', *Journal of Behaviour and Experimental Psychiatry*, 12, 1981, 241–47.

17. Davies, A.D.M. and Snaith, P.A. 'The Social Behaviour of Geriatric Patients at Mealtimes: An Observational and an Intervention Study', *Age and Ageing*, 9, 1980, 2, 93–9.

18. Langer, E.J. and Rodin, J. 'The Effects of Choice and Enhanced Personal Responsibility for the Aged: A Field Experiment in an Institutional Setting', *Journal of Personality and Social Psychology*, 34, 1976, 191–8.

19. Rodin, J. and Langer, E. 'Long Term Effects of a Control-relevant Intervention', *Journal of Personality and Social Psychology*, 35, 1977, 12, 897–902.

10 TREATMENT: THE USE OF MEDICATION, AND LEGAL CONSIDERATIONS

Many years ago doctors used to devise their own prescriptions. The symbol used for prescribing, ℞/H5, stands for 'recipe' and many early prescriptions were individual concoctions of various substances. Now, with a wide range of active and standardised drugs, the art of prescribing lies more in choosing the right preparation or combination of drugs. The emphasis on effective pharmacology has, however, tended to detract from another aspect of prescribing; the non-pharmaceutical one. Years ago rich patients might have received the advice to go on a cruise or to one of the spas 'for the waters' or to a mountain or seaside resort 'for the air'. Just as we now have a better understanding of pharmacology, we also have a better understanding of the psychological and social principles of non-pharmaceutical treatment. This has been dealt with in earlier chapters. Here we deal with some of the principles and some of the problems of prescribing medication for old people.

Some of the Problems

One British multi-centre study of nearly 2,000 admissions to geriatric facilities found over 80 per cent of patients were on prescribed drugs. Nearly 250 of those patients were suffering from adverse reactions and in over 200 cases adverse reactions had contributed to the need for admission. Anti-hypertensive drugs, anti-Parkinsonian drugs, psychotropic drugs and especially diuretics, were the most important groups causing adverse reactions.[1] Another study reported nearly 15 per cent of admissions to a psychogeriatric unit were suffering direct effects of psychotropic medication, including behaviour disturbance, hypotensive episodes and excessive sedation.[2] Castleden has stated that there is an exponential increase in adverse reactions and a linear increase in non-compliance with increasing numbers of drugs prescribed.[3] Nor, of course, are all drugs taken prescribed. Many can be bought 'over the counter' at chemist's shops or drug stores. Elderly women in the UK are, for example, often avid consumers of laxatives! Alcohol is another commonly consumed drug with many interactions with prescribed drugs.[4] Whilst psychotropic drugs can cause physical side effects, drugs prescribed for physical disease can also cause psychiatric symptoms. Anticholinergic drugs such as benzhexol are sometimes prescribed for Parkinson's disease and have been shown experimentally to impair memory in old people.[5] L-dopa, bromocriptine and other anti-Parkinsonian drugs can also cause psychotic reactions. Many anti-hypertensive drugs may cause psychiatric problems.[6] Propanolol can cause behavioural disorder, hallucinations and paranoid psychosis; methyldopa and clonidine sleep disorders; propanolol and methyldopa delirium, depression and even apparent cognitive impairment.

Prescribing for old people rarely seems to be logical. One general practice study in the UK showed that 50 per cent of patients over the age of 65 years were receiving repeat prescriptions. On review 62 per cent of these were classed as essential, 28 per cent of these as equivocal and 10 per cent as definitely unjustified.[7] Another study of over 1,000 repeat prescriptions showed that the longer repeat prescribing continued the less likely it was to be monitored and the more likely the patient was to be elderly.[8] In view of all these problems it is necessary to review the basic facts of drug use in old people.

Drug Handling

Discussions of drug handling usually begin with *absorption*. When dealing with old people, it is important to remember two preliminary steps, getting and taking (see Figure 10.1). *Getting* a prescription filled out is not at all easy for old people. Sadly, doctors on home visits sometimes write a prescription and give no thought as to how the patient will actually obtain the drugs prescribed. Sometimes a friend, neighbour or voluntary organisation can help, sometimes the doctor needs to arrange to pick up the prescription himself or ask another professional to help. Often, if the patient can be tided over the first few days with an initial supply given by the doctor, that will give time for someone to get to the local chemist's shop.

Taking medication is not always that easy. Some old people find childproof safety containers impossible to open.[9] Often the bottles are not labelled in a way that is comprehensible to the patient. Large-print labels with simple, clear instructions are essential. Explaining the medication to the patient, ideally with the tablets in hand for demonstration, is the best way of ensuring that they are taken properly.[10] If drug regimes are complicated, or if the patient is depressed or mildly confused, noting down the purpose of the tablets and when they should be taken

Figure 10.1: Steps in the Handling of Drugs

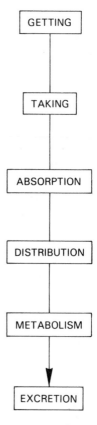

on a large card, with samples sellotaped to the card if necessary, can clarify things. Alternatively, for some people, drug drawers which enable a day's medication to be laid out in individually 'timed' drawers can be of benefit. Most important, it must never be assumed that, because a drug has been prescribed, it has been taken. Patients sometimes suffer adverse effects when they move into hospital or an old people's home and suddenly start to take drugs which have been prescribed in increasing doses because of apparent ineffectiveness at home which was really due to the patient not taking the drugs. Depot injections, although not ideal for old people for many reasons, are sometimes the only way of ensuring that chronic schizophrenic patients get their medication.

Absorption

This is the first stage in the conventional metabolism of drugs. It may be slowed by a full stomach or by competition with other drugs. So far, differences in absorption have not been consistently demonstrated between old and young people.

Distribution

The ratio of lean to fatty tissue decreases with ageing. Many drugs are distributed selectively in lean or fatty tissue. Alcohol is a good example of this and experimental work has shown that after intravenous infusion of a dose of alcohol standardised for body area, old people achieve higher peak serum concentration, largely because of increased body fat.[11] Lowering of plasma albumin in ill old people can result in greater availability of drugs which are usually protein-bound.

Sensitivity

Target organ sensitivity is only beginning to be explored. The way in which hypokalaemia affects the sensitivity of the heart to digoxin has been known for some time but the question of the sensitivity of the various brain receptors to psychotropic drugs and how this varies with age is largely unanswered, although it has been suggested that such increased sensitivity may be the mechanism for the decrease in the intravenous sedative dose of diazepam with increasing age.[12]

Metabolism

Most drug metabolism is carried out in the liver. Differences have been found with a slowing of oxidation of chlormethiazole, for example, in some old people. On the other hand, oxidation of some of the benzodiazepines is not impaired. Interactions occur here too. Heavy smoking and alcohol consumption induce enzymes speeding metabolism of some drugs. Old people are generally not heavy smokers or drinkers and enzyme induction does not usually occur unless provoked by another prescribed drug. Anti-epileptic drugs can sometimes interfere with each other in this way. Liver damage through chronic alcohol abuse produces impaired metabolism. It is important to remember this, for example, when treating withdrawal symptoms in alcoholism with chlormethiazole. Plasma half-life, the time it takes for a drug to decline to half of its peak level, is a rough measure of metabolism. For many benzodiazepines, this is doubled in old age. This can bring major problems of accumulation with drugs such as nitrazepam, leading to 'hangover',[13] confusion, unsteadiness and falls. Many drugs (e.g. chlorpromazine) have active metabolic products which make assessment of their handling extremely complicated.

Excretion

Renal function may be impaired in old age. Many drugs or their metabolic products depend on renal excretion for elimination. Some of these can themselves lead to renal impairment. In psychiatry, lithium is the classical example of a drug which is excreted unchanged by the kidneys and where minor upsets in renal function can lead to accumulation and further compromise of renal function with the risk of a potentially fatal vicious circle.

Adverse Effects

Interactions

The potential for drug interactions is higher in old people because they are such heavy consumers of prescribed drugs. *The British National Formulary*[14] has tables of interactions and no attempt will be made to reproduce those here. A few examples will be given to illustrate the problems. Tricyclic antidepressants and beta-blocking drugs cause postural hypotension. When given together, there can be a profound synergism of these side effects rendering the patient incapable of standing up without fainting. Case 4.4 is an example of this. Diuretics interact with lithium, reducing excretion and causing a risk of potentially fatal toxicity. Patients on lithium should not normally be given diuretics. If treatment with both drugs is essential, it should be very carefully monitored. Not all interactions are harmful. Patients with resistant depression, unresponsive to tricyclic antidepressants alone, sometimes respond to tricyclic antidepressants together with lithium. In the confused patient who is very disturbed at night, a combination of neuroleptic and hypnotic may sometimes prove a more effective night sedation with less hangover effect than either drug alone.

Side Effects

Many psychotropic drugs have *anti-cholinergic* actions. In some neuroleptics like chlorpromazine and thioridazine, the inbuilt anticholinergic effects help to neutralise the tendency of the primary action of the drug, dopamine blockade, to cause Parkinsonian symptoms. Anticholinergic side effects generally include dry mouth, blurred vision, constipation and impaired memory. Severe anti-cholinergic side effects such as glaucoma and urinary retention are relatively rare but important.

Dopamine blockade by neuroleptic drugs occasionally causes an acute dystonic reaction. This resembles the occulogyric crisis of post-encephalitic Parkinsonism. The patient's head is suddenly thrown violently back, then there is a phase of relaxation, after which the process may be repeated. This rare reaction is sometimes seen after a single dose of a neuroleptic and once seen is never forgotten. It can be aborted by a dose of intra-muscular or intravenous procyclidine. More common but slower to develop is the Parkinsonian syndrome with slowing of movements (bradykinesis), loss of associated movements (e.g. arm swinging when walking), tremor (characteristically a pill-rolling tremor, made worse by emotional arousal) and cogwheel rigidity. The best way of treating this is to keep neuroleptic medication to the minimum needed by the patient to live as independently as possible. In elderly schizophrenic patients, a dose of neuroleptic sufficient to suppress symptoms fully will often render the patient completely immobile and so a suitable compromise between therapeutic and side effects has to be sought. The use of anti-cholinergic drugs to routinely suppress symptoms caused by neuroleptic drugs is to be deprecated in old people because anti-cholinergic drugs bring their own side effects, already mentioned. The longest-term side effect of neuroleptic treatment is tardive dyskinesia. Restless oro-facial movements with lip-smacking, tongue-rolling and gum-chewing are the commonest symptoms of tardive dyskinesia but larger muscle groups may also be involved. Oro-facial dyskinesia can often be made worse by ill-fitting dentures. Tardive dyskinesia is an unpleasant side effect that only fades very slowly if the neuroleptic is stopped. There is little effective treatment for it, though it may be temporarily suppressed by increasing neuroleptic dosage. It is best to avoid this complication as far as possible by limiting long-term neuroleptic treatment to those patients for whom it is essential. While neuroleptic drugs are associated with resting and postural tremors, lithium and anti-convulsants tend to produce an action tremor.[15]

A Personal Pharmacopoeia

There are three main groups of drugs in psychiatry: the neuroleptics, the antidepressants (including lithium) and the minor tranquillisers. It is best to learn a few drugs in each group thoroughly. A personal pharmacopoeia of favourite drugs is enumerated below. This list is far from comprehensive and reflects personal experiences and preferences. For a more comprehensive view, the reader is referred to the *British National Formulary* and other appropriate texts. A short discussion of electroplexy (ECT) is included in this section.

Neuroleptics

Thioridazine. This is probably the neuroleptic of choice for symptomatic control of the behaviourally disturbed old person. It *does not* treat confusion; indeed its sedative and anti-cholinergic effects may worsen confusion. Long-term high dosage use has occasionally been linked with the serious complication, retinitis pigmentosa. Promazine is another drug with a similar profile of action.

Haloperidol. This is an effective neuroleptic for controlling acutely disturbed patients. It is a specific and effective treatment for schizophrenia. It has little anti-cholinergic effect and therefore readily induces extrapyramidal side effects. It does not usually cause postural hypotension. There is a very rare but potentially disastrous interaction with lithium.[16] This produces an encephalitis and occasionally irreversible brain damage. *Trifluoperazine* has a similar profile of action to haloperidol, but seems to be less sedative. Interactions with lithium are not reported.

Chlorpromazine. This is also highly effective but more sedative, more likely to cause postural hypotension, more anti-cholinergic and therefore less likely to cause extrapyramidal problems than haloperidol or trifluoperazine.

Flupenthixol Injection. If a long-acting neuroleptic injection is needed for the chronic schizophrenic patient, this seems to be the best compromise between efficacy and side effects. It does have extrapyramidal side effects and so dosage should be kept to a minimum. Often 20 to 40 mg intra-muscularly every two or four weeks will suffice. The oral preparation of flupenthixol is said to have antidepressant properties and sometimes low-dose intra-muscular flupenthixol is used as an adjuvant treatment in chronic depression. This is not an approved indication but will sometimes increase the co-operativeness of the negativistic patient enabling oral antidepressants to be given more readily. Clopenthixol, a relatively sedative but related drug, is useful for the over-active patient who needs a more sedative depot injection. Depot injections should not normally be used in the demented patient.

Antidepressants

Dothiepin. This seems to retain the effectiveness of the older tricyclics such as amitriptyline and imipramine with less of the side effects. It still has relatively strong anti-cholinergic and sedative effects and the majority of the daily dose should be given at night. In order to minimise side effects, it is also usual to increase dosage gradually. In overdose, it is, like other tricyclics, cardiotoxic and should be used with caution in people with known arrythmias.

Mianserin. This is probably the best proven of the 'newer' non-tricyclic antidepressants. It has less cardiotoxic and anti-cholinergic effects than the tricyclics. Like dothiepin, it tends to be sedative and there tends to be a two to three week delay between starting treatment and mood improvement. The patient should always be warned about side effects and about the delay before beneficial effects are likely to be experienced. Mianserin sometimes cause joint and muscle pain and causes bone marrow suppression in rare instances.[17]

Lithium Carbonate. Especially effective in manic-depressive and recurrent depressive illness, this drug has a low therapeutic margin and serum levels which should run at around 0.4 to 1.0 twelve hours after the last dose must be carefully monitored, initially weekly and eventually fortnightly or monthly. Good renal function is an essential prerequisite to treatment[18] and thyroid function should be checked every few months as this is sometimes suppressed. Twice daily dosage is preferred to a single daily dose. Sometimes patients who do not respond to dothiepin, mianserin or lithium alone will respond to another antidepressant or to a combination of dothiepin or mianserin with lithium. Patients on lithium should be warned about the risks of toxicity and told to stop the treatment immediately if they develop nausea, diarrhoea, vomiting or if they are otherwise unwell. They should report this immediately to their doctor who can advise them when to re-start their medication. Printed cards with a warning about side effects and toxicity are available, and can be very useful (Figure 10.2).

Phenelzine. This drug of the mono-amine oxidase inhibitor class can be effective in patients with mixed anxiety and depressive symptoms. It calls for dietary and drug restrictions and the patient should be told about these and should always carry a warning card. Its effect in appropriate subjects is dramatic but, once started, the treatment is very hard to withdraw without relapse.

Figure 10.2: Example of a Lithium Treatment Card

Lithium Treatment Card

ALWAYS CARRY THIS CARD WITH YOU

If you become ill from whatever cause and require a doctor please show him this card.

Name...

Address...

....

Clinic...

Telephone...

Doctor...

Lithium is a treatment used to prevent excessive mood swings, and to be effective must be taken regularly. Remember that you should continue taking your tablets as your doctor directs even though you feel perfectly well.

The following notes are for your guidance:—

1. Take the tablets regularly at the same time each day as directed by your doctor. The dose has been selected individually to suit you.

2. The dose may need adjusting in the first few weeks of treatment and this is judged by your blood test results. On the day of your blood test do not take your tablets until after the test.

3. Like most medicines, lithium carbonate may have some 'side effects'. Usually these will last only for a short time.

4. Tell your doctor at once if you have any of the following:—
   diarrhoea or vomiting
   giddiness or loss of balance
   abnormal drowsiness
   severe trembling of hands or feet
   excessive thirst
   increased urination.

5. The doctor will want to see you from time to time to check your progress and to make sure that your dose remains correct.

The reverse of this card carries a table with spaces for appointments, dose of lithium and serum levels.

Minor Tranquillisers

Diazepam. One of the earliest benzodiazepines and one of the cheapest, this drug has an extended half-life in old people and dosage should be kept very low. Generally drugs of the benzodiazepine group are best avoided in old people. If relaxation is needed, it should be provided by appropriate social or psychological therapy (Chapter 8), rather than by drugs. Diazepam also has an occasional use in very severely demented patients with muscle spasm where its muscle relaxant effects can be useful.

Lormetazepam. At present, this seems to be one of the best hypnotics for old people. It is a small tablet, easy to take and has an intermediate half-life with little hangover or cumulative effect providing dosage is kept low. Nitrazepam is best avoided in old people because of risks of accumulation and temazepam is harder to take than lormetazepam, sometimes too short-acting with wakening in the middle of the night and, occasionally, seems to produce the need for increasing dose and a risk of dependency. All the benzodiazepines carry this risk to a greater or lesser degree and in patients who have been receiving them for some time, they should be discontinued gradually, to avoid withdrawal symptoms.

Chlormethiazole. A non-benzodiazepine tranquilliser, this is an effective night sedative and can be used to reduce daytime agitation in confused patients, especially those who react adversely to a neuroleptic such as thioridazine. It is available either in capsule or liquid form. The patient may find the liquid preparation rather unpleasant-tasting although this can sometimes be disguised with orange juice.

Electroplexy (ECT)

This is the treatment of choice for severely depressed patients, especially if life is threatened by dehydration or suicide. Unilateral non-dominant treatment twice weekly is less likely to cause memory problems.[19] In any case, for most patients memory problems are transient and less severe than those caused by the depression itself. The patient is anaesthetised and given a muscle relaxant to modify the fit. It is essential that ECT is followed by a period of antidepressant or lithium therapy to minimise the risk of relapse. Because of 'bad press', ECT is probably given less appropriately than it should be at present.

It must be stressed again that the above is a brief list of the treatments most commonly used by one of the authors. It is not intended to be exhaustive and many details such as dosage, interactions and some side effects, have been omitted. The list emphasises that a relatively small group of drugs can cover most psychiatric situations and that the latest is not necessarily the best.

The Principle of Minimal Medication

Stated briefly, this principle is that old people should always be given the minimal amount of medication necessary to treat their illness or alleviate their suffering. Alternatives to drug treatment should always be sought. A good example of this is the patient who complains of insomnia. This may be symptomatic (e.g. early morning wakening in depressive illness or paroxysmal nocturnal dyspnoea in heart failure) and, if so, it should be treated appropriately. On the other hand, the patient may simply have unrealistic expectations. Total amount of sleep needed seems to decrease with increasing age,[20] especially if the patient takes little exercise and 'catnaps' through the day and the patient may not realise this. Practical non-pharmaceutical measures should precede any use of medication. More exercise, more interesting activity during the day, excluding 'catnaps' and the traditional warm milky drink at night can all be tried. On the other hand, if the patient is drinking too much in the afternoon and evening, especially if the drinks contain stimulants like caffeine or diuretics like caffeine and alcohol, then sleep may be interfered with by over-stimulation or the need to rise repeatedly to go to the toilet and drinking may have to be restricted. Management of insomnia in the confused patient has been discussed briefly in Chapter 5 and illustrated in Figure 5.4. Another common symptom that responds better to rational analysis than symptomatic prescribing is incontinence, Case 10.1 illustrates this.

Case 10.1:
  B.Y. was a 93-year-old widow who lived alone in an old back-to-back terraced house. Her mobility had become restricted and she had started to sleep in her downstairs room which was a combined living room and kitchen. Her toilet was down two flights of outside stairs in the cellar. She became incontinent because of difficulty in reaching the toilet and a commode was provided but she refused to use it, saying that it did not flush and was in her kitchen. She was referred to the psychogeriatric service because of confusion and incontinence. She

had mild intellectual impairment but fairly logical reasons for not using the commode. When admitted to day hospital, she behaved quite appropriately and went to the toilet and used it readily. Because of a multitude of problems, her adjustment at home was very poor and she has now been admitted to hospital to await urgent residential care. Her incontinence was almost entirely situational in cause.

The case of B.Y. illustrates how important environmental factors are in the causation and management of incontinence. Equally a local cause such as urinary infection, retention (possibly caused by drugs) or severe constipation may be responsible for incontinence. Only when these and other causes have been excluded should a symptomatic pharmacological approach be considered.

The symptomatic use of drugs, for example the use of neuroleptics to control disturbed behaviour or a hypnotic at night, should be distinguished from their specific use (e.g. neuroleptics for schizophrenia or antidepressants for depression). When drugs are being used symptomatically, it is especially important to seek alternatives and limit the length of treatment. When drugs must be used, then the principle of minimal medication states that the following rules apply: the *smallest possible number* of drugs should be used at any one time to reduce the possibility of harmful interactions. The *smallest effective dose* should be used. The drug should be prescribed for the *shortest time* necessary for effective treatment. The principle of minimal medication is summarised in Table 10.1.

Table 10.1: The Principle of Minimal Medication

1	Seek alternatives
2	Distinguish specific from symptomatic treatment
3	Give the smallest number of drugs
4	In the lowest effective dose
5	For the shortest time needed

This chapter stresses the risks of careless prescribing. It cannot be emphasised too much that pills are only part of the doctor's therapeutic armamentarium. In conjunction with other disciplines, psychological and social help can and should be offered when appropriate. Using a neuroleptic to sedate a confused elderly patient at home or on a long stay ward because service inadequacies lead to under-stimulation is little different in principle to the abuse of psychotropic drugs to control political dissenters in some countries. Both involve the use of chemical agents to hide or compensate for social deficiencies. Doctors should not fall into this trap. However, we must not over-react against drugs. We must remember that, properly used, psychotropic drugs can cure illness, alleviate suffering and even save life. A further discussion of drug treatment for the elderly mentally ill can be found in the *Handbook of Geriatric Psychopharmacology*.[21]

The Law in Relation to Treatment

American and United Kingdom law and practice in relation to mental health and compulsory treatment show interesting differences. United Kingdom law is encapsulated in the Mental Health Act (1983)[22] which has been explored in some detail by Bluglass.[23] Two strands can be detected in both United Kingdom and American legislation. The first is the necessity to protect others from someone else's madness. This had been described as a sort of 'policing' function. The second is the need to protect the interest of the mentally ill person against exploitation and to ensure that mentally ill people receive appropriate treatment whether or not they consent to this. This can be described as a kind of 'parental' function. In England and Wales, the Vagrancy Acts of 1713 and 1744 allowed the detention of the mentally ill who might be dangerous on the order of two or more justices and the Madhouses Act of 1744 tried to ensure minimum standards in private institutions. Thus the two strands of legislation can be seen even at that early date. In the United Kingdom, the Mental Health Act (1959) firmly moved the care of the mentally disordered away from the judicial into the medical sphere (except when a crime had been committed). This tradition has been thankfully maintained in the Mental Health Act (1983) though the Mental Health Review Tribunals of a quasi-judicial nature have been introduced to give patients a right of appeal against their detention.

In the UK the question of patients' capability of handling their own affairs is dealt with quite separately from the question of detention and compulsory treatment under the somewhat archaic institution of the Court of Protection.

In the USA where litigation and lawyers are much more frequently encountered than in the UK, judicial procedures have been retained although 'competency' and 'commitment' hearings are no longer linked. Each state has its own mental health code. Some states even have a 'bill of rights' for inpatients including a 'right' to 'the best quality of care'. The presence of a legal framework does not of itself ensure quality of care and the UK system deals with these questions of quality of care through an advisory administrative machinery, the Health Advisory Service, recently supplemented by the Mental Health Commission of the 1983 Act. American legislation appears to be going through many changes and the section on the law in the *A Comprehensive Textbook of Psychiatry*[24] questions whether the trend in the USA to medicalise deviant behaviour is now being replaced by a tendency to criminalise the mentally ill. United Kingdom and American law also differ on their interpretation of the question of consent to treatment. In the USA 'informed' consent is the term used to cover the patient's right to know all about the likely effects and risks of treatment. The UK legal concept of consent ('real' consent) allows the doctor discretion to decide exactly how much information to give to the patient; the doctor still has a duty to inform the patient but the extent of this information is to be judged by what would be regarded as good medical practice and not by some absolute duty to disclose everything.

The authors of this text are only familiar with United Kingdom legislation and the remainder of this discussion will be devoted to this. A fuller explanation of United Kingdom legislation can be found in Bluglass[23] and of American legislation in the relevant section of *A Comprehensive Textbook of Psychiatry.*[24]

The Mental Health Act of 1983 has sections that deal with compulsory admission for assessment (Section 2, Section 4 in emergency) and for treatment (Section 3) as well as enabling a voluntary patient who is already receiving treatment for mental illness to be detained in hospital (Section 5) for up to 72 hours to enable a Section 2 or Section 3 to be implemented.

Section 2

Section 2 is the standard means of compelling a patient to go into hospital for a period of up to 28 days' assessment (which can include necessary treatment). An application must be made by a social worker or the patient's (legally defined) nearest relative. Two medical recommendations are necessary, one normally from a doctor who has known the patient for some time (usually the general practitioner), the other from a doctor approved by the Secretary of State for Health under Section 12 of the Mental Health Act as having special experience in the diagnosis and treatment of mental disorders (usually a consultant or senior registrar in psychiatry). In their recommendations the doctors must state that the patient is suffering from mental disorder of a nature or degree that warrants detention in hospital and that compulsory admission is necessary in the interests of the patient's health or safety or for the protection of other persons. The patient and his nearest relative, when possible, must be informed of the implementation of the Section and of rights of appeal. There are carefully defined rights of appeal to specially-set-up Mental Health Review Tribunals and the hospital managers also have the ability to discharge a patient. The responsible consultant or the nearest relative may discharge the patient from the section at any time but the responsible doctor can block the relative's right of discharge under certain circumstances. Once the papers have been completed, the social worker has the right to take steps to convey the patient to a hospital which has agreed to accept him. A representative of hospital managers (usually a senior nurse) must formally receive the patient and the papers.

Section 4

Section 4 depends on the medical recommendation of only one doctor and is only to be used in an emergency if undue delay would result from seeking a second opinion. The use of this section has to be justified and explained on the relevant legal document. It lasts for only 72 hours, otherwise in most respects it is similar to Section 2.

Section 3

Section 3 is a treatment section (although necessary treatment may also be given under Section 2). It again requires two medical recommendations although they must be more detailed in this case. The application can be made by a social worker but in this case the nearest relative's consent is essential. In exceptional circumstances, the nearest relative can be displaced by legal action. Section 3 lasts initially for six months. Specific treatments (presently only psychosurgery and the surgical implementation of hormones) can only be given with the patient's consent *and* the approval of a Mental Health Tribunal. Other treatment (for example, ECT) can only be given without the patient's consent if a second opinion from a Mental Health Act Commissioner supports this. The nearest relative, as well as the responsible medical officer, has the right of discharge although again the relative's right can be blocked in certain circumstances by the responsible medical officer. The patient must be informed of his rights including rights of appeal. A particular line of treatment cannot be continued beyond three months without the patient's consent or the support of a second opinion from a Mental Health Act Commissioner.

Section 5(2)

Section 5(2) enables the responsible medical officer or his named deputy to detain a previously voluntary patient in hospital for up to 72 hours whilst a Section 2 or Section 3 is implemented. Section 5(4) is a holding power for designated senior nurses which can only be implemented if a patient is already receiving treatment for mental disorder, only extends for six hours and is only used when it is not practicable to secure the immediate attendance of a medical practitioner to implement Section 5(2).

Court Orders

Other parts of the Mental Health Act enable the courts to remand patients to hospital for report on their mental condition, to remand them to hospital for treatment and to make interim hospital orders so that the offender's response in hospital can be evaluated without irrevocable commitment to this method of dealing with the offender if it should prove unsuitable. These court powers are rarely used with old people and will not be discussed in any detail here.

The Mental Health Legislation and the Demented Patient

When is Detention Detention? The common-law duty of care means that when looking after confused patients staff have to take reasonable precautions against them wandering off and coming into danger. A 'confusion lock' (usually a door with two handles, both of which have to be operated simultaneously) is as big an obstacle to some demented patients as a mortice lock to the mentally well. It would, however, be extremely cumbersome and expensive to put every demented inpatient on a Section 2 or Section 3 and would be against the spirit of successive Mental Health Acts which have sought to reduce rather than increase the need for compulsory detention. Most doctors prefer to treat their demented patients informally except under very special circumstances. Nurse staffing levels can be highly relevant here as informal care is often possible with an adequate number of nurses whereas a shortage of nurses is more likely to lead to the need for locked doors.

Consent. Many demented patients in hospital do not understand where they are and almost by definition they are unable to understand treatment or give fully informed consent in the same way that a person who was mentally well or indeed suffering from another form of mental illness might be able to. It is considered essential under the Mental Health Act that formally detained patients who cannot give consent should have their treatment reviewed at three months by a Mental Health Act Commissioner. Should not the same standard also apply to informally treated patients with dementia who are not able to fully understand their treatment? This is a hard question. Its answer hinges on the interpretation of 'consent'. UK law has so far taken the view that the doctor can exercise his professional judgement in deciding how much information should be given to a patient in seeking to obtain consent, and has adhered to the concept of real consent. The potential expense and bureaucracy of over-eager application of the Mental Health Act is enormous and health professionals, especially doctors and social workers, have to perform a delicate balancing act between their patient's 'right to consent' and what is reasonable and in the patient's best interests.

The Court of Protection and Power of Attorney

In England and Wales a power of attorney becomes invalid when patients become incapable of managing their own affairs. This is not always appreciated and relatives sometimes continue to exercise a power of attorney when it is legally invalid. The Law Commission[25] has recently issued a report recommending that an 'enduring' power of attorney should be available in England and Wales as it is in Scotland and some other countries. This would enable a person when mentally well to provide for someone else to manage their affairs when they became mentally incapable. The Law Commission has recommended that, subject to certain safeguards, legislation should be enacted to enable an 'enduring' power of attorney to be used in England and Wales. At present, however, the only alternative for management of a demented patient's affairs is the Court of Protection which can be unduly cumbersome and expensive, especially if only small amounts of money are involved. Application to the court is usually made through a solicitor and may be made by a solicitor or a doctor or other interested person. Usually the application is made by a near relative of the mentally ill patient. The Court of Protection requires a medical report and serves notice on the patient, through his doctor, that a court 'hearing' will be held at a specified time and place. Following this hearing, a receiver is appointed to look after the patient's affairs under the supervision of the Court of Protection. The court was originally set up to manage a relatively small number of cases and is in danger of being swamped by the volume of work with the increasing number of demented old people.

Many relatives exercise financial control over the affairs of demented patients in a less formal way (for example, through authorities to draw cheques on the patient's bank account). These authorities have often been issued early in the course of the patient's illness when they were able to make some judgement about such matters and relatives do not always appreciate that they are technically no longer valid when the patient becomes unable to exercise control over their own affairs. Although the legal status of such powers is dubious and they cannot be recommended, in many cases they do seem to be a reasonable way of managing the patient's affairs, at least to those exercising them. The law in this area needs clearing up and legislation for an 'enduring' power of attorney would be one way of doing this.

Conclusion

The emphasis of this book has been on the practice rather than the theory of psychiatry with old people. We have tried to cover these practical aspects thoroughly and to give appropriate references for those who wish to pursue them. Our aim has been to show that proper psychiatric care of mentally ill old people is immensely worthwhile and rewarding. We have pointed to political issues as well as purely psychiatric issues as we believe that proper care for old people is dependent upon the political will and economic commitment to provide it. We hope that you have found the book useful and thought-provoking.

Notes

1. Williamson, J. and Chopin, J.M. 'Adverse Reactions to Prescribed Drugs in the Elderly: A Multi-centre Investigation', *Age and Ageing, 9*, 1980, 2, 73–80.

2. Briant, R.H. 'Drug Treatment in the Elderly: Problems and Prescribing Rules', *Drugs*, 13, 1977, 225–9.

3. Castleden, C.M. 'Prescribing for the Elderly', *Prescriber's Journal*, 18, 1978, 4, 90–4.

4. Anonymous leader, 'Drugs and Alcohol', *British Medical Journal*, 1980, 1, 507–8.

5. Potamianos, G. and Kellett, J.M. 'Anthicholinergic Drugs and Memory: The Effects of Benzhexol on Memory in a Group of Geriatric Patients', *British Journal of Psychiatry*, 140, 1982, 470–2.

6. McClelland, H.A. 'Psychiatric Reactions to Antihypertensive Drugs', *Adverse Drug Reactions Bulletin*, 1983, 99, 364–7.

7. Tulloch, A.J. 'Repeat Prescribing for Elderly Patients', *British Medical Journal*, 282, 1981, 1672–5.

8. Dennis, P.J. 'Monitoring of Psychotropic Drug Prescribing in General Practice', *British Medical Journal*, 1979, 2, 115–16.

9. Sherman, F.T., Warach, J.D. and Libow, L.S. 'Child Resistant Containers for the Elderly', *Journal of the American Medical Association*, 241, 1979, 10, 1001–2.

10. Macdonald, E., Macdonald, J.B., Phoeni, M. 'Improving Drug Compliance After Discharge', *British Medical Journal*, 1977, 2, 618–21.

11. Vestal, R.E., McGuire, E.A., Tobin, J.D., Andres, R., Norris, A.H. and Mezey,

R. 'Aging and Ethanol Metabolism in Man', *Clinical Pharmacology and Therapeutics*, 21, 1977, 3, 343–54.

12. Cook, P.J., Flanagan, R. and James, I.M. 'Diazepam Tolerance: Effect of Age, Regular Sedation and Alcohol', *British Medical Journal*, 289, 1984, 351–3.

13. Cook, P.J., Huggett, A., Graham-Pole, R., Savage, I.T. and James, I.M. 'Hypnotic Accumulation and Hangover in Elderly Inpatients: A Controlled Double-blind Study of Temazepam and Nitrazepam', *British Medical Journal*, 286, 1983, 100–2.

14. *The British National Formulary* (British Medical Association and the Pharmaceutical Society of Great Britain, No. 9, London, 1985).

15. Lane, R.J. 'Drugs and Tremor', *Adverse Drug Reaction Bulletin*, 1984, 106, 392–5.

16. Thomas, C.J. 'Brain Damage with Lithium and Haloperidol' (letter), *British Journal of Psychiatry*, 134, 1979, 552.

17. Page, C.E. 'Mianserin Induced Agranulocytosis', *British Medical Journal*, 284, 1982, 1912–13.

18. Hansen, H.E. 'Renal Toxicity of Lithium', *Drugs*, 22, 1981, 461–76.

19. Fraser, R.M. and Glass, I.B. 'Recovery from ECT in Elderly Patients', *British Journal of Psychiatry*, 133, 1978, 524–8.

20. Quan, S.F.B., Bamford, C.R. and Beutler, L.E. 'Insomnia', *Geriatric Medicine*, 15, 1985, 1, 11–15.

21. Jenike, M.A. *A Handbook of Geriatric Psychopharmacology* (PSG Publishing Company, Littleton, Mass., 1985).

22. *The Mental Health Act 1983*, Her Majesty's Stationery Office, London.

23. Bluglass, R. *A Guide to the Mental Health Act* (Churchill Livingstone, London, 1983).

24. Kaplan, H.I. and Sadock, B. *A Comprehensive Textbook of Psychiatry*, 4th edn (Wiliams and Williams, Baltimore, 1985).

25. The Law Commission, *The Incapacitated Principal* (July 1983, Her Majesty's Stationery Office, London, No. 122, Cmnd 8977).

GENERAL FURTHER READING

Arie, T. (ed.) *Recent Advances in Psychogeriatrics,* (Churchill Livingstone, Edinburgh, 1985)

Birren, J.E. and Sloane, R.B. (eds) *Handbook of Mental Health and Aging,* (Prentice Hall, Englewood Cliffs, 1980)

Isaacs, A.D. and Post, F. (eds) *Studies in Geriatric Psychiatry,* (J. Wiley, Chichester, 1978)

Kay, D.W. and Burrows, G.D. *Handbook of Studies on Psychiatry of Old Age,* (Elsevier, Amsterdam, 1984)

Levy, R. and Post, F. *The Psychiatry of Late Life*, (Blackwell Scientific Publications, Oxford, 1982)

Lishman, W.A. *Organic Psychiatry*, (Blackwell Scientific Publications, Oxford, 1986)

Pitt, B. *Psychogeriatrics*, (Churchill Livingstone, Edinburgh, 1982)

INDEX